A COLOUR ATLAS OF
PAEDIATRICS

General Editor, Wolfe Medical Atlases:
G. Barry Carruthers, MD(Lond)

Copyright © M. Dynski-Klein, 1975
Published by Wolfe Medical Publications Ltd, 1975
Printed by Smeets-Weert, Holland
ISBN 0 7234 0184 5
4th impression 1982

This book is one of the titles in the series of
Wolfe Medical Atlases, a series which brings
together probably the world's largest systematic
published collection of diagnostic colour
photographs.
For a full list of Atlases in the series, plus
forthcoming titles and details of our surgical,
dental and veterinary Atlases, please write to
Wolfe Medical Publications Ltd, Wolfe House,
3 Conway Street, London W1P 6HE

Tralee General Hospital Library

This book must be returned not later than the last date stamped below.

FINES WILL BE RIGOROUSLY IMPOSED

30. JUL 200		

A colour atlas of
Paediatrics

MARTHA DYNSKI-KLEIN

MD (Prague), MRCS, LRCP, DCH (London)

Honorary Consultant Paediatrician, West Middlesex Hospital
Late Deputy Chief, University Children's Clinic and
Paediatric Consultant
University Clinic for Obstetrics and Gynaecology, Prague

WOLFE MEDICAL PUBLICATIONS Ltd

Acknowledgements

Most of the photographs have been taken by Mr D A Vinten, medical photographer-in-charge at the West Middlesex Hospital, and his staff to whom I wish to express my sincere thanks for their co-operation and skill. Likewise I thank Miss S Robinson, the medical artist, for her accurate drawings (**138**, **375** and **376**).

I am indebted to Dr D Morley for permission to publish **160**, **254**, **256**, **258** and **259**, and Mr M Stranc for the photographs shown in **46**, **47** and **116–118**, to Mr I Bierer, Mr D Stern and the late Mr C W F Burnett, Consultant Obstetricians, for their interest and the acceptance of the paediatric invasion into the obstetric stronghold, and to Sisters M Gatenby, I Ròdgers and M C Pattison for their devoted help.

Thanks also to Professor G H Valentine for permission to reproduce two chromosome preparations (pages 312 and 314) from his book *The Chromosome Disorders* (Heinemann Medical Books).

My gratitude is due to Professor A Howe for his valuable advice and criticism of the manuscript, to Mrs S Raphael for her competent secretarial assistance and especially to my dear husband for his unfailing encouragement and constructive help in the preparation of this Atlas.

Finally, I wish to thank the publishers for their courtesy and excellent presentation.

Martha Dynski-Klein

To Pepi, Hermann and the child patients

CONTENTS

Introduction

'While I have eyes to see'.
(*Hesperides,*
Robert Herrick, 1591-1674)

A picture, it is said, is something between a thing and a thought. Language on its own is often inadequate to describe medical phenomena satisfactorily. Pictorial presentation enhanced by colour is a very impressive medium which will help the reader to become conversant with his subject.

Faced with the patient, the visual recollection of the relevant clinical signs will facilitate the planning of appropriate investigations to verify a spot diagnosis. Pictorial follow-up throughout the formative years may reveal the influence of inborn developmental trends and the effect of treatment on the course of diseases. The Atlas has been compiled with this purpose in mind.

With few exceptions the material has been collected by the author from cases in the Paediatric Department and in the Newborn and Premature Unit of the West Middlesex Hospital.

The photographs are arranged chronologically, corresponding to the stages of infancy, childhood and puberty, and are subdivided into sections as found in standard textbooks to enable the association of the illustrations with the text.

Some entities, mainly of genetic origin and the complexities of chromosome aberrations, are presented in a special chapter. Miscellaneous conditions of practical significance are contained in a separate section and in the Appendix.

In view of the longterm approach some cases may appear or be referred to in different chapters, and some relevant conditions are shown in more than one case where individual variations need to be demonstrated.

The presentation of rarities has not been the foremost intention. The reader will find that emphasis has been laid on developmental and nutritional problems, genetic disorders and especially on neonatal conditions, where observation and evaluation of signs and symptoms has to replace verbal communication with the patient. Attention is drawn to normal phenomena, to deviations from the norm and particular features important for the differential diagnosis.

The legends to the photographs are necessarily concise and limited to the description of leading signs, whilst clinical facts are mentioned only where essential for the basic understanding of the case. The reader should have no difficulty in complementing his knowledge by looking up suitable textbooks.

Considering the wide field of paediatrics, comprehensiveness cannot be claimed. Many conditions do not show up well in still photography and not all afflictions have entered the hospital gates.

It is hoped this Atlas will provide a representative pictorial cross-section of paediatric conditions to guide and stimulate the student and assist the interested physician.

The Newborn and the First Trimester

This is the most crucial period of childhood. Research covering this age group has been motivated by the awareness that the medical and social measures for the care of mother and child introduced since the turn of the century have dramatically reduced the high infant morbidity and mortality rate without comparable beneficial effect in the first three months of life.

A new approach had to be sought and resulted in the evaluation of factors harmful to the foetus during its intra-uterine existence, to the baby at delivery and during the perinatal period. The search has been enhanced by the daring methods of intra-uterine investigations (*amniocentesis* and *amnioscopy*), by biochemical advances and by the rapidly expanding knowledge of genetic cytology and chromosomal aberrations. A sophisticated machinery monitors the baby throughout the critical phases of intra-uterine development and birth, demanding close co-operation of the obstetric and paediatric personnel and appropriate institutional facilities.

There is concern that by these efforts lives may be saved which would become a severe burden to family and society. However, as all these measures are aimed at an *intact survival* the hazard is lessened by the antenatal diagnosis of disabling genetic and other diseases, and the knowledge of the recurrence risk. Appropriate counselling and family planning should forestall the procreation of unwanted life.

For the postnatal period a comprehensive screening programme has been evolved which will reveal, apart from other diseases, inborn metabolic disorders. Early nutritional therapy can prevent progressive neurological damage and other physical disabilities.

An essential part of the programme is the assessment of the infant's development and condition. An intimate knowledge of the unique and multiform manifestations of this age group is imperative for adequate care.

NORMAL APPEARANCE AND FUNCTIONS

1 A mature newborn Delivery was spontaneous at 40 weeks' gesta-tion. The skin is bright red and covered with *vernix caseosa*, a foetal product of the sebaceous glands, shed cells and hair. The eyes are closed ; the limbs are held in foetal flexure position. The creases visible on the left palm and the acrocyanosis of the perioral area and lower part of the extremities are normal.

2 Normal well-set ear and mature plantar creases Two plastic clamps compress the cord. This technique ensures a firm grip.

3 A different technique of cord ligation employs a rubber band which gradually shrinks with the cord.

4 A 7-day-old infant The flexure posture of the limbs is still main-tained. The cord has separated. There is a small granuloma on its base. If there is discharge of urine or faecal material a persistent, patent urachus or an omphalomesenteric fistula is present which should be excised.

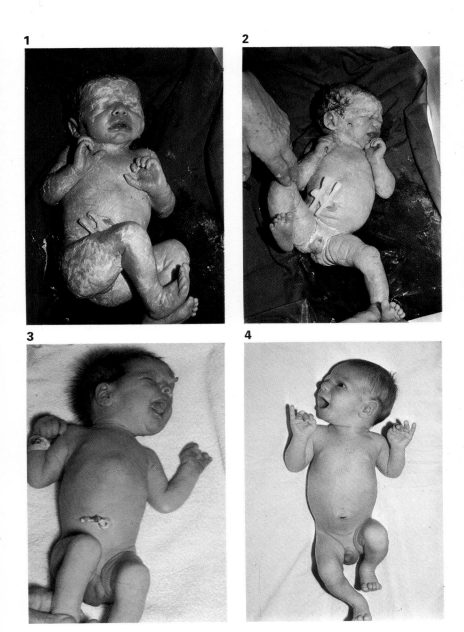

Automatic reflexes (5-12) are signs of primitive neuromuscular response to stimulation. With normal development most of these reactions fade out within the first trimester.

5 & 6 Attempts at primary creeping in semi-prone position, and (**6**) primary creeping with crossed legs.

5

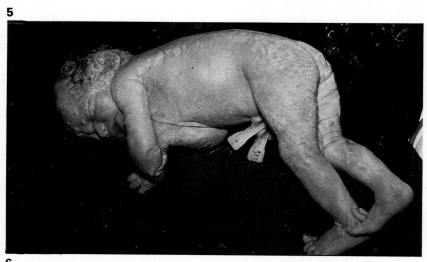

6

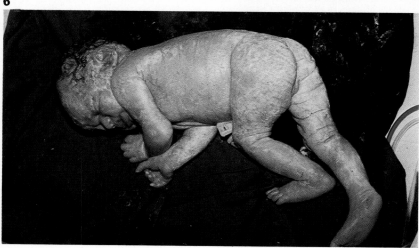

10

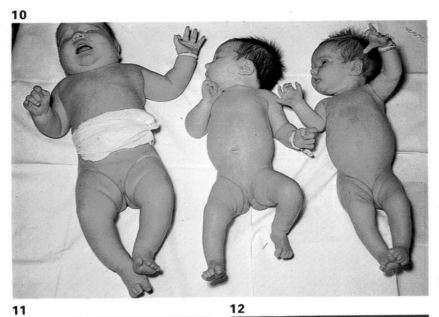

11

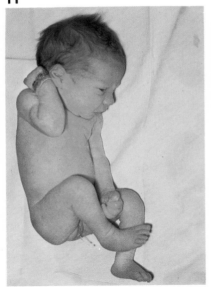

12

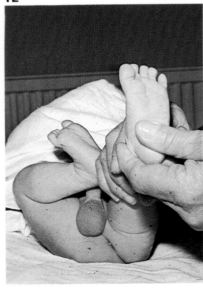

Other signs distinctive for the newborn (13-24)

13 Muscular hypotonus of the back muscles causes sitting kyphosis and absence of the cervical and lumbar lordosis.

14 Muscular hypertonus Leg extension is limited in the *'heel-to-ear'* manoeuvre. Note the popliteal angle of approximately 90°

15 Sucking pads on both lips with callus formation engorge during sucking, enabling a firm grip on the breast.

13

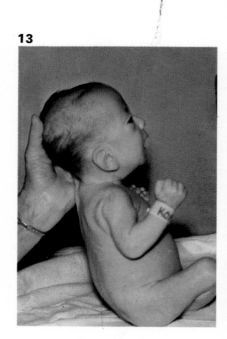

14

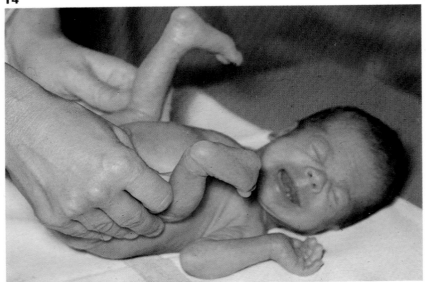

15

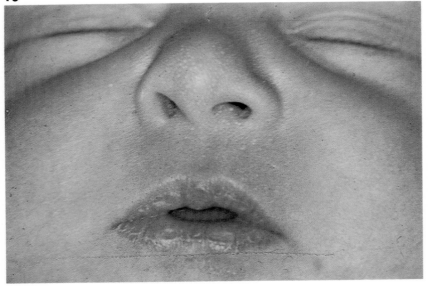

16 Sucking cushions Pads of fat tissue between the fibres of the masseter muscle prevent the indrawing of the cheeks when sucking. The fat tissue remains unaltered by weight loss.

17 Another sucking aid The serrated membrane on the alveolar ridge swells and strengthens the grip of the gums.

18 Epstein's epithelial pearls (Bohn's nodules) A cluster of epithelial inclusion cysts on the raphe of the hard palate. Not to be mistaken for monilia patches.

19 Retrognathia A benign transitory condition without functional disability.

20 Milia White papules on the tip of the nose are hyperplastic sebaceous glands, the effect of maternal transplacental hormones. They disappear with desquamation.

16

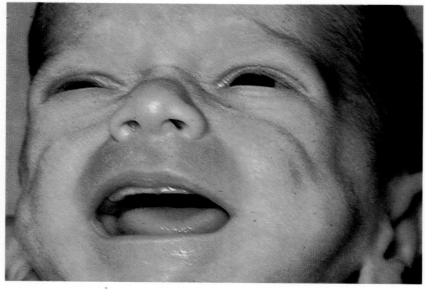

17

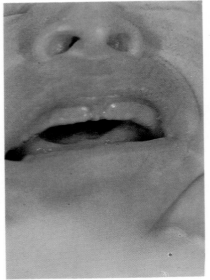

18

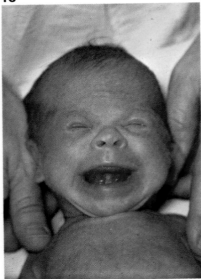

19

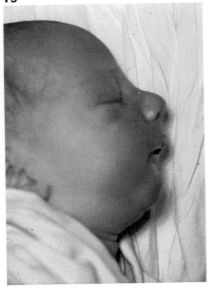

20

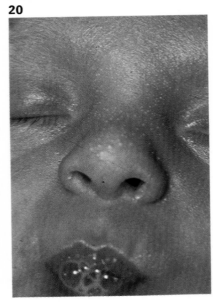

21 & 22 Erythema toxicum of the newborn A benign, self-limiting common phenomenon of erythematous, maculo-papular or vesicular character. Eosinophilia and the presence of eosinophils in the vesicles indicate the allergic aetiology (**21**). The rash becomes confluent and intensified in areas subject to irritation (**22**).

23 & 24 Physiological desquamation Paper-thin peeling. The skin beneath is healthy. This process is more marked in areas of irritation.

21

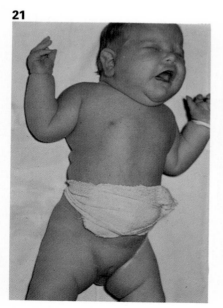

22

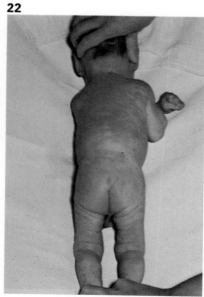

23

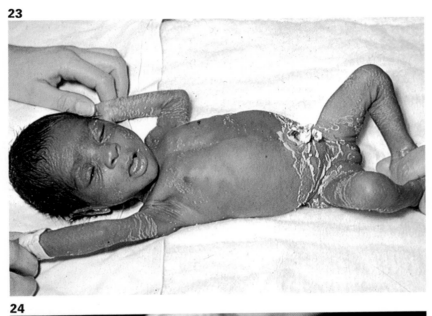

24

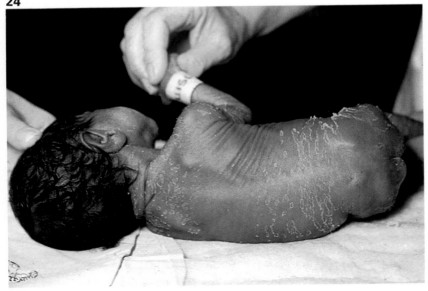

VARIATIONS OF APPEARANCE
AND FUNCTIONS

25 A shocked baby delivered by caesarian section for foetal distress. Note the marked acrocyanosis. The frog-like position is due to transitory hypotony.

26 Other signs of cerebral irritation There is absence of the plantar grasp and a positive Babinski reflex, extension of the big toe.

27 A 'floppy' baby in 'frog-like' position The development of stance is often delayed in these babies (*see* **619**).

28 'Heel-to-ear' manoeuvre in an abnormal hypotonic infant. There is no resistance to leg extension and the popliteal angle is absent.

25

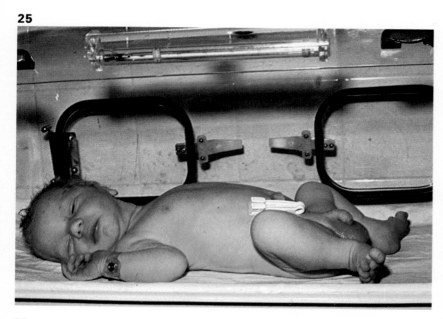

26

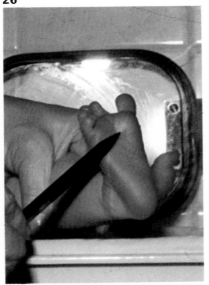

27

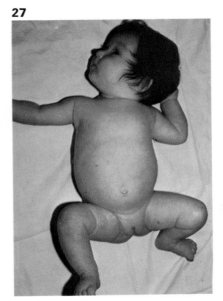

28

29 Overstretching of ligaments after frank breech delivery with extended legs. Recovery will be complete.

30 General hypotonus ('rag-doll' baby) in an infant with brain damage.

31 General hypertonus with extensor spasm of the limbs and neck retraction as seen in kernicterus (*see* **200**).

29

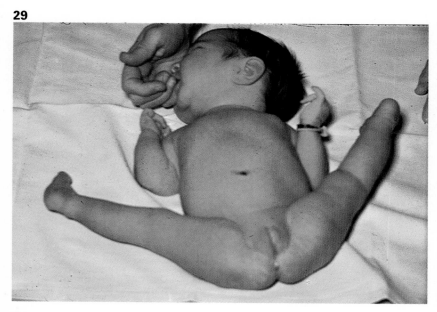

30

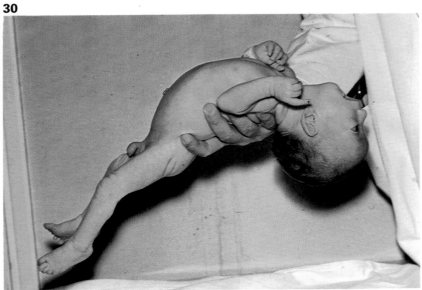

31

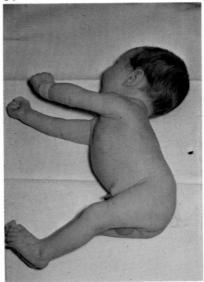

32 & 33 Natal teeth Buds of dental tissue may appear with other malformations. The baby has microcephaly, hirsutism, severe micrognathia and malformed ears.

34 Micrognathia in an otherwise well-developed baby. The mandibular hypoplasia improves with development.

35 Micrognathia of severe degree may produce sucking and breathing difficulties especially in a premature baby (*see* **539**).

32

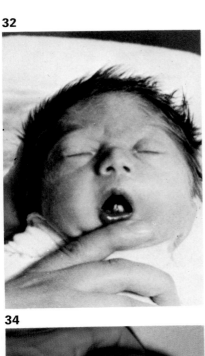

33

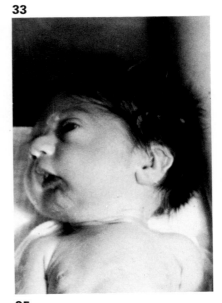

34

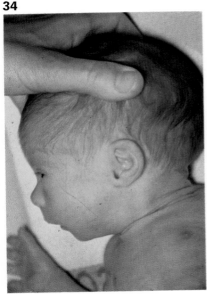

35

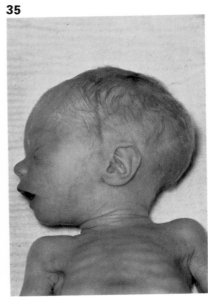

Birthweight and size correlate with gestational age and development. Infants deviating from the normal pattern face increased perinatal risk because of their liability to obstetrical and postnatal complications.

36 'Small-for-date' hypoplastic baby born at 38 weeks' gestation. Weight and length are below the 3rd centile for gestational age. The mother was a heavy smoker, a condition associated with intra-uterine retardation of foetal growth.

37 'Light-for-date' baby born at 43 weeks' gestation. The baby shows signs of intra-uterine malnutrition due to insufficiency of an infarcted placenta. The length is normal for gestational age, but the weight was below the 3rd centile. The shrivelled face and loose skin indicate acute intra-uterine weight loss.

38 Extremes The gestation of the preterm baby was interrupted at 33 weeks (*appendicectomy in the mother*). The infant was developmentally normal for gestational age; birthweight 1170g. The macrosomic baby of 39 weeks' gestation shows the condition associated with intra-uterine overnutrition in maternal diabetes; birthweight 6360g.

36

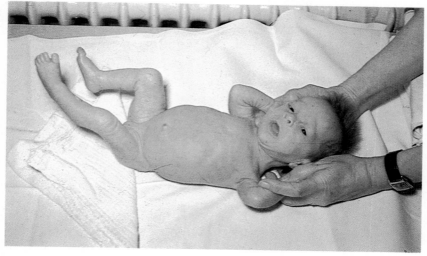

37

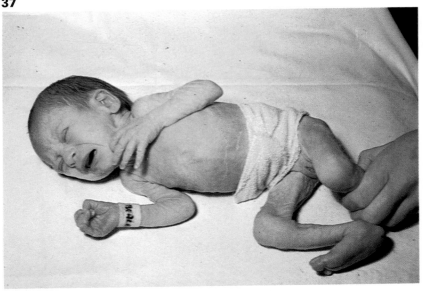

38

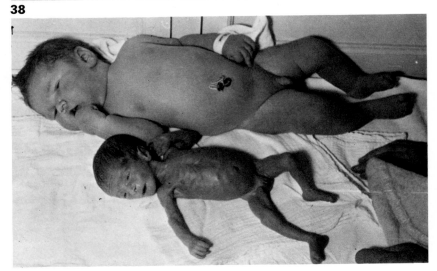

Birthmarks are common skin disorders, usually of transitory nature.

39 & 40 Naevi flammei Distended capillary vessels are seen on the forehead, eyelids, philtrum, chin and nape of neck. They usually disappear during the first year.

41 Vascular naevi simulate mottling of the skin. They involute gradually.

39

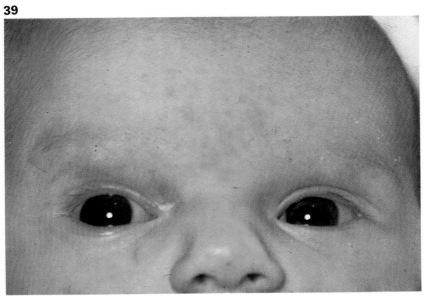

40

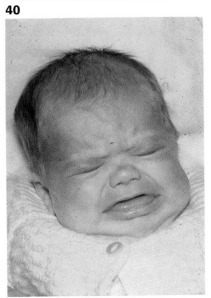

41

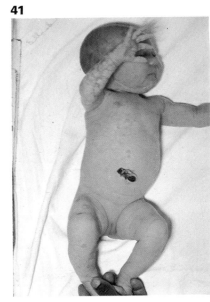

42 Port-wine stain naevus in the area of the first division of the trigeminal nerve. These naevi are permanent and are often part of cerebral angiomatosis (*see* **547-549**).

43 Large deeply-pigmented 'bathing trunk' naevus A permanent condition which could develop later into melanoma.

44 Mongolian spots are circumscribed blue-grey pigmentations in the lumbar area due to an accumulation of dopa-positive melanocytes, more common in coloured infants. Note also *neonatal lanugo*.

45 Mongolian spots in a white baby along the spinal tract. They should not be mistaken for bruises (*see* **586 & 587**).

46 A large, irregularly shaped skin defect on the trunk.

47 Appearance 4 years later with successful plastic reconstruction.

42

43

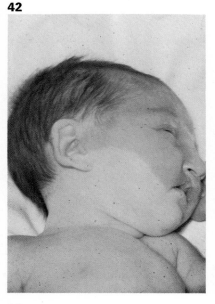
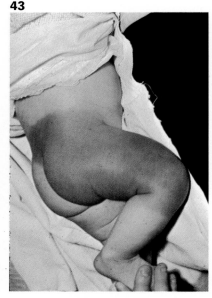

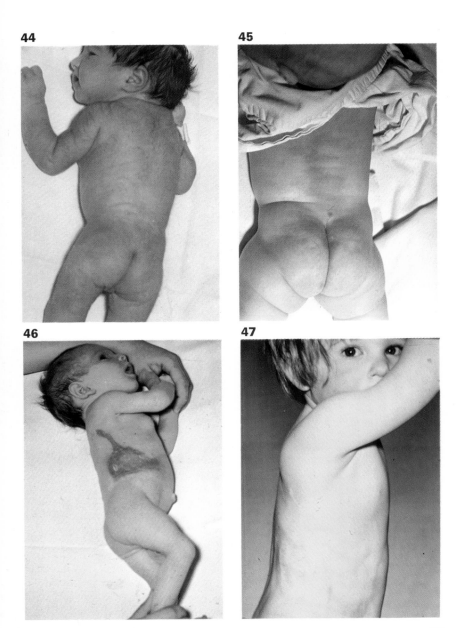

48 Congenital skin defect on both knees Sharply defined rectangular areas are denuded of all layers of skin.

49 Close-up of 48 shows granulations on the base of the defect and raised hyperaemic edges.

50 After 4 weeks the areas are covered by a thin translucent atrophic membrane. Elastic fibres are absent, in contrast to normal scar tissue.

48

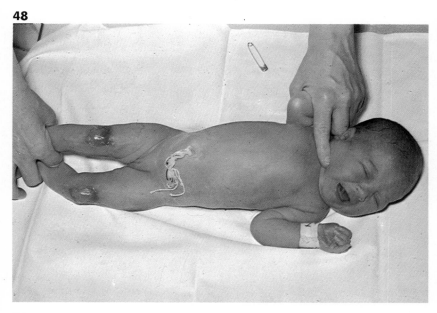

49

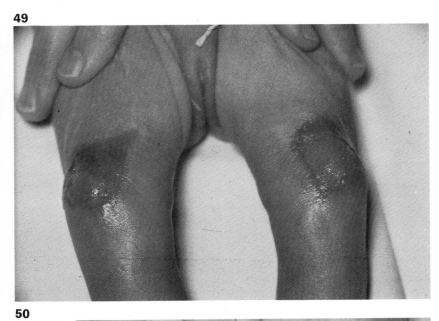

50

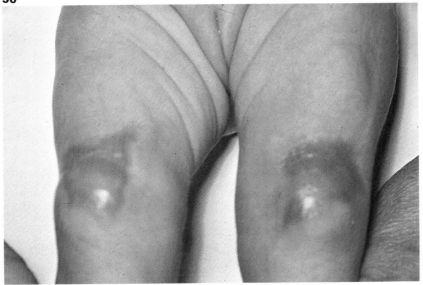

BIRTHTRAUMA

Many injuries are of transitory character. Advances in obstetric practice and perinatal care are reducing the incidence of permanent damage.

HEAD INJURIES

51 Bruising of the face following face presentation. The nasal septum is deflected. Initially this may produce sucking difficulties.

52 Puffiness of the face and petechiae The cord was twisted around the neck.

53 Moulding and overriding of the skull bones occurs to some degree normally during delivery. Here the high ridge of the parietal bones overlapping the frontal ones and the sagittal suture indicates disproportion and a difficult delivery.

54 Spoon shaped depressed skull fracture results from pressure of the sacrum in pelvic disproportion. Intracranial injury may occur. Note the low-set abnormally shaped ear.

51

52

53

54

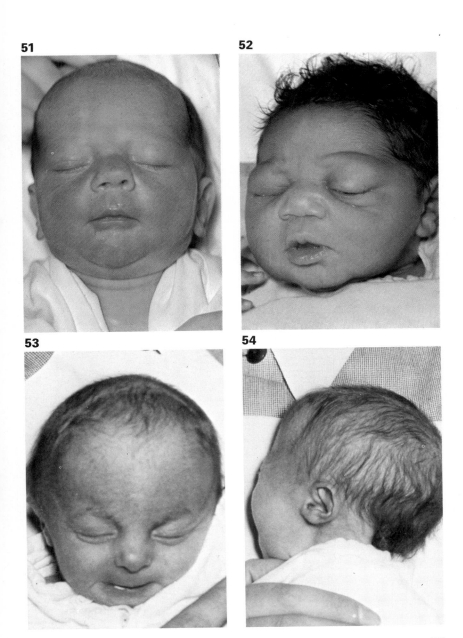

55 Caput succedaneum A short-lasting, ill-defined oedema of the presenting part. The location indicates the intra-uterine lie of the foetus.

56 Unilateral cephalhaematoma The subperiostal bleeding is limited by the firm adhesion to the sutures.

57 Bilateral cephalhaematoma The effusion is divided by the firm attachment of the periosteum to the sagittal suture. Gradual resorption occurs within a few weeks.

55

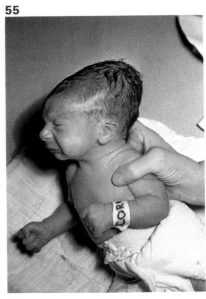

56

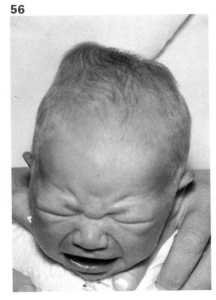

57

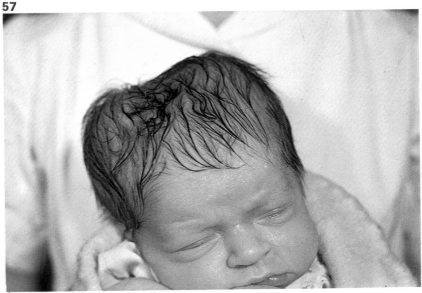

58 Pyo-cephalhaematoma Pyogenic infection developed after tapping. An unnecessary procedure.

59 Necrosis of the scalp over the crown and parietal bones due to pressure and ischaemia during prolonged labour (*observed also in the trisomy 13 syndrome*).

60 Close-up shows the deep pressure marks corresponding to the sutures, and the intense swelling and necrosis.

58

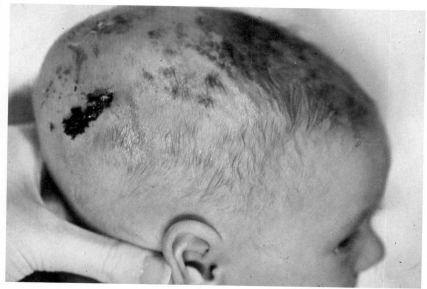

59

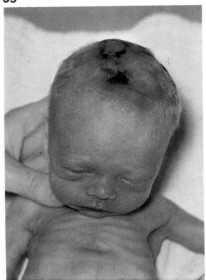

60

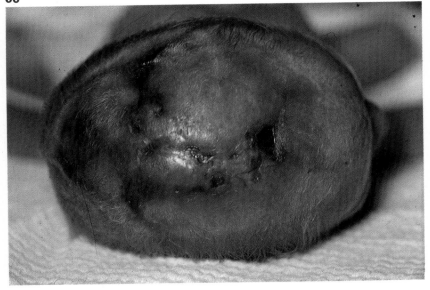

61 'Sign of the setting sun' A transitory phenomenon in prematures and infants suffering from birth shock. It is elicited by a quick change of the baby's position from the supine to the upright, indicating cerebral irritation and midbrain dysfunction. The upper eyelid is retracted, and the iris is partly covered by the lower eyelid, giving the appearance of a sunset. Note the *blue sclerae* and the normal *red reflex*.

62 In severe brain damage this sign is persistent (*see* **485**).

63 Visus hydrocephalicus A similar phenomenon, here the result of shallow orbits and depression of the eyeballs by increased intracranial pressure.

61

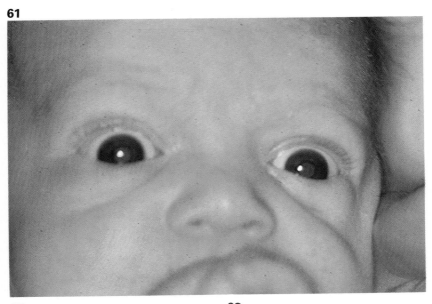

62

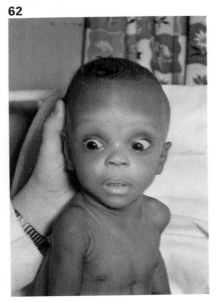

63

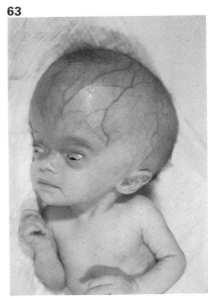

64 Cerebral oedema following rapid delivery The infant shows signs of cerebral irritation, retracted neck, arched trunk and accentuated flexure posture. The child survived with *minimal brain damage*.

65 Intracranial haemorrhage Baby seen in a tonic convulsion. Note trunk and neck retraction, rotation and extensor spasm of the crossed legs. The baby died during a convulsion.

64

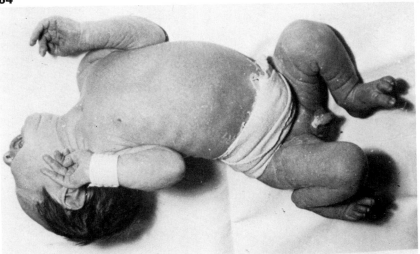

65

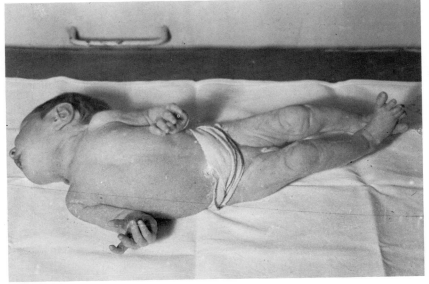

PERIPHERAL NERVE INJURIES

66 Lower brachial plexus root injury (Klumpke-Déjerine) and facial nerve paralysis following a difficult breech delivery. There is claw-hand formation by flexion of wrist and fingers of the right hand. On the left side the eye cannot be closed, the naso-labial folds are flattened and the mouth is drawn to the healthy side.

67 Horner's syndrome Injury to the sympathetic fibres within the anterior roots of the first and second thoracic segment. May appear together with the above injury. There is ptosis, enophthalmos and contraction of the pupil of the left eye.

68 'Wrist drop' in radialis paralysis Note the necrotic patch on the right upper arm, the result of intra-uterine pressure and ischaemia. Normal function did return.

69 Pseudo 'wrist drop' seen in a 'floppy', hypotonic baby.

66

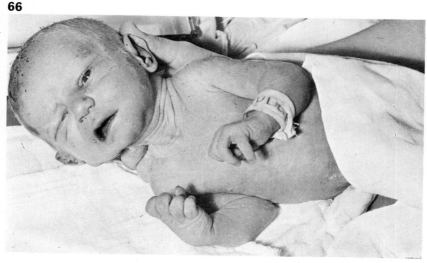

67

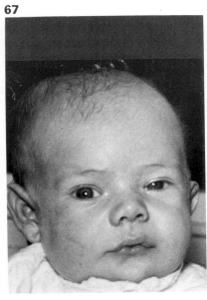

68

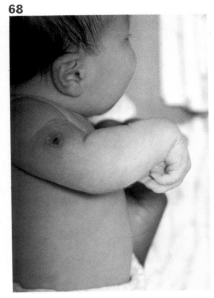

69

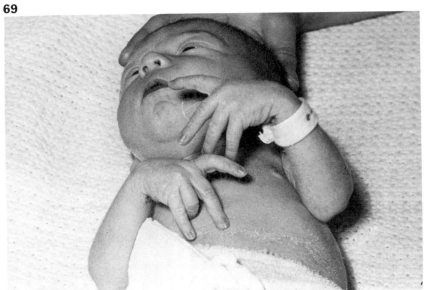

70 Supination is not disturbed in this condition.

71 Torticollis The head is tilted, due to shortening of the sterno-mastoid muscle. Results from spasm or haemorrhage and fibrosis. The left-sided facial palsy affects mainly the depressor muscle of the lower lip (*top, left*). These signs are intensified by crying (*top, right*). Three months later (*bottom, left*) the function of the first and second nerve branch is normal. The mouth branch has still not fully recovered. At the age of 5 months (*bottom, right*) the head is held straight, but the left angle of the mouth is still drawn to the right. If persistent, supranuclear agenesis of the nerve or a congenital defect of the depressor anguli oris muscle exists. The white patch on the tongue is due to *thrush* (*monilia*) infection.

70

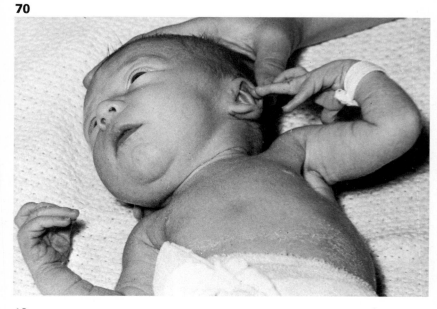

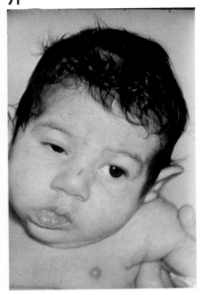
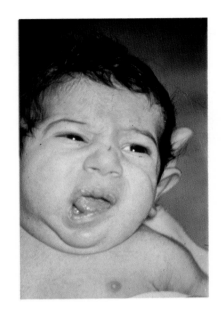
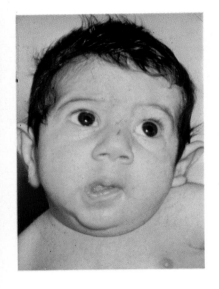
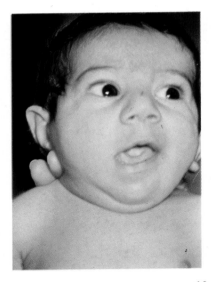

METABOLIC DISTURBANCES

72 Neonatal hypoglycaemia producing convulsions. A transient metabolic disturbance. Blood sugar was below 20mg/100ml. The mother had toxaemia of pregnancy. Routine testing of the blood sugar is part of the neonatal screening programme.

73 Neonatal hypocalcaemic tetany with carpal spasm (*main d'accoucheur*). This state of relative hypoparathyroidism with low calcium and high phosphate blood levels is accentuated by concentrated cow's milk feeding. Maternal hyperparathyroidism is found in some instances.

72

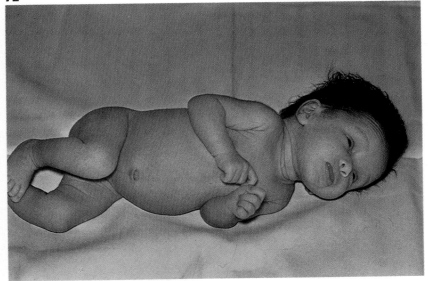

73

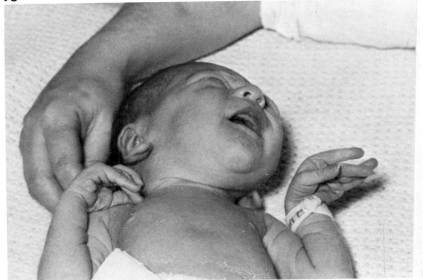

CONGENITAL MALFORMATIONS

CORD AND UMBILICUS

74 Haemorrhagic cysts within the amnion sheet of the cord. A rare abnormality associated with other malformations ; here with amputation deformity of the left hand (*see* **108**).

75 Partial exomphalos, a severe form of early developmental retardation of the abdominal wall. The baby shows penial haemorrhage and *holoprosencephaly*. Note the abnormal flexure of the fingers of the right hand as seen in trisomy 18 E1 (*see* **137, 439** *and* **570, 571**).

76 Close-up shows the intestinal coils in the translucent sac which consists of amnion and peritoneum (*see* **137**).

Immediate surgical repair, which may be difficult, is now successfully replaced by 'tanning' the sac with mercurochrome. After epithelisation the resulting hernia needs surgical repair.

74

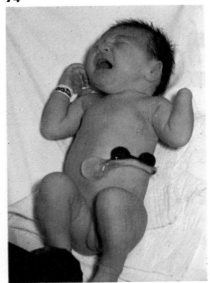

75

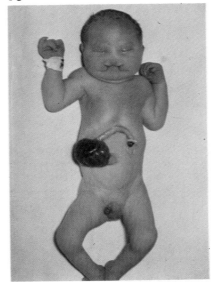

76

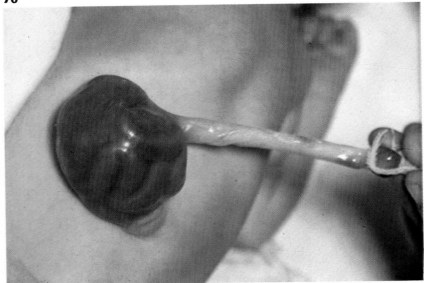

77 Large umbilical hernia A less severe form. The sac is covered by normal skin and contains various amounts of viscera. Prevalent in coloured infants. Spontaneous retraction occurs to a considerable degree.

78 Umbilical hernia of a more common size The hernia is easily reducible.

79 Cutis (skin) navel The hard stump is the remnant of the cord covered with skin. Not reducible, in contrast to hernia.

80 Divarication (diastasis) of the recti muscles A developmental retardation, frequently connected with prematurity. Improves with maturation.

77

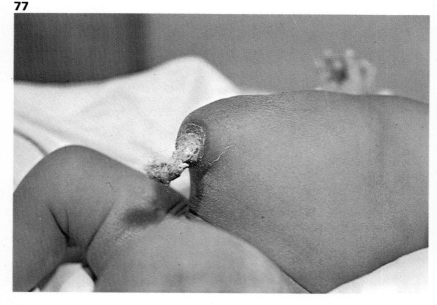

78

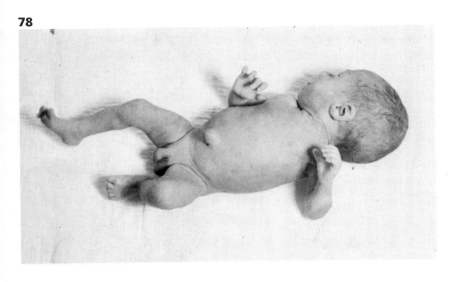

79

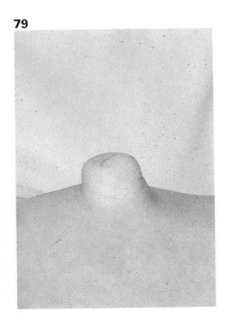

80

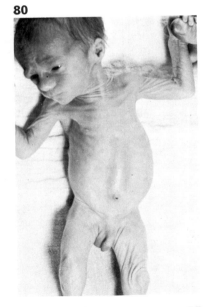

CRANIOSYNOSTOSIS

81 Scapho (dolicho) cephaly caused by premature closure of the sagittal suture. Prevalent in males. Intracranial pressure signs are usually absent.

82 Oxy (acro) cephaly results from early closure, partial or total, of the coronal suture. The deformity frequently appears with other anomalies. Intracranial pressure develops early, leading to exophthalmos and brain damage (*see* **520-527**).

83 Craniolacunia (Lückenschädel) The intra-uterine x-ray picture shows the characteristic *honeycomb* skull. This malformation is usually connected with spina bifida. Note the deformity of the vertebrae in the mid-thoracic region.

81

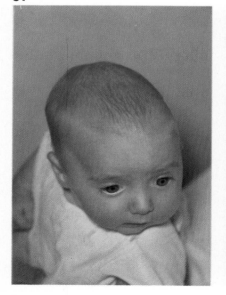

82

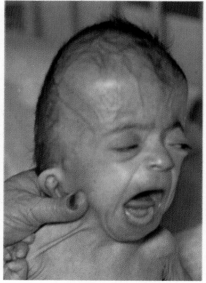

83

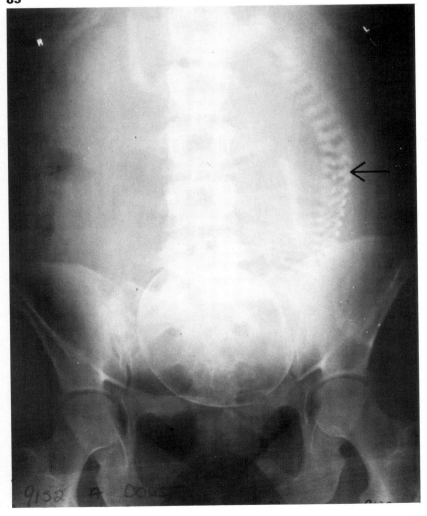

THE NEURAL PLATE

84 Congenital hydrocephalus results from overproduction, defective absorption or obstruction of the circulation of cerebrospinal fluid. Early neurosurgical treatment is indicated to prevent further brain damage.

85 Hydrocephalus before (*left*) and after (*right*) ventriculo-atrial shunt operation via insertion of the *Spitz-Holter valve*.
   The shunt has to be maintained for life. Normal intellectual and neuromuscular function might be achieved if progression is halted. During early childhood regular revision is necessary to prevent shunt failure.

84

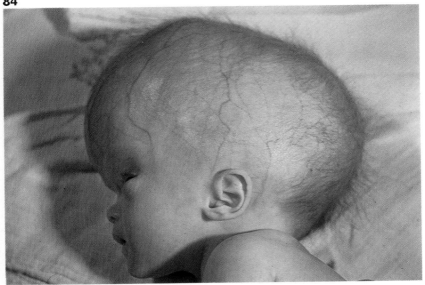

85

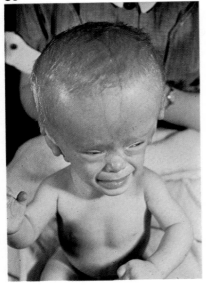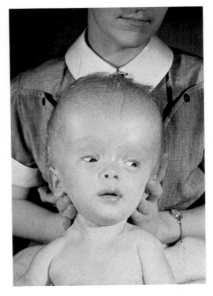

Failure of closure defects appear as sinuses and cystic deformities of variable severity.

Sinuses (86-88) are epithelium-lined defects extending from the skin into the neural canal. When patent they act as portal of entry for infections and should be excised.

86 Cranial-dermal sinus, usually situated in the midline of the occiput.

87 Pilonidal sinus A common deformity. The distal end of the neural tube is attached to the coccyx.

88 Spinal-dermal sinus, may occur anywhere along the spinal canal.

86

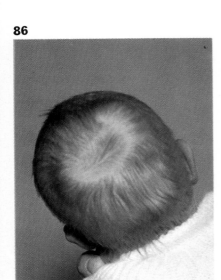

87

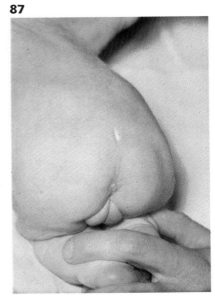

88

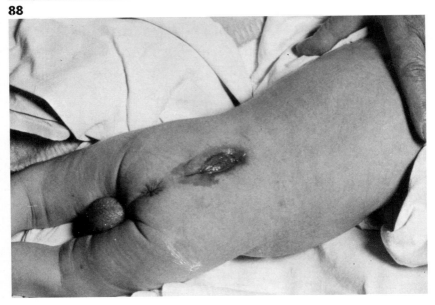

Cystic deformities (spina bifida cystica) (89-102) appear as meningoceles and myelomeningoceles.

Meningoceles contain mainly meningeal tissue and are usually not connected with functional disability. Immediate neuro-surgery will prevent perforation and infection.

89 Lumbo-sacral meningocele This is the most frequent localisation.

90 Cervical meningocele covered by a translucent vascular membrane and skin.

91 & 92 Another case The sac remained intact during birth, but perforated soon afterwards.

93 Cranial-meningo-encephalocele fluctuates in size according to changes of the intracranial pressure (e.g. enlarges by crying or coughing).

89

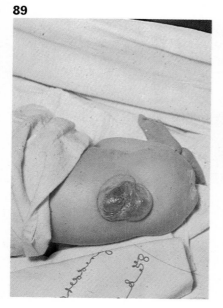

90

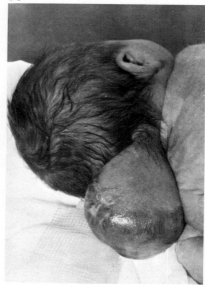

91

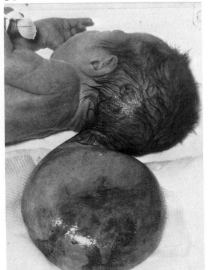

92

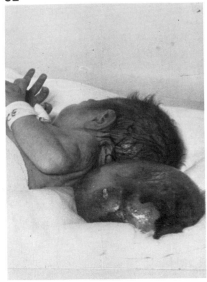

93

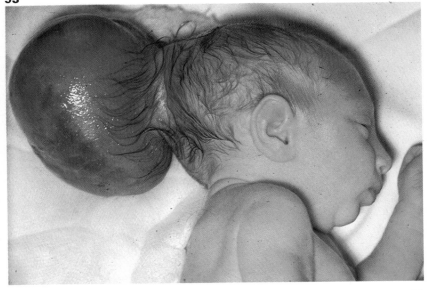

Myelomeningoceles are always connected with disability. The sac contains meningeal and neural tissue. The 'quality of life' and survival rate is influenced by the level of the neurological lesion. Highly situated lesions have the worst prognosis.

These cases illustrate the dilemma and controversy surrounding the selection for surgical therapy.

94 Thoracic myelomeningocele Severe disability ensued.

95 & 96 Thoraco-lumbar myelomeningocele with Arnold-Chiari phenomenon The brainstem and cerebellum are displaced into the cervical canal. The sac is covered with skin and a vascular membrane. Note the large hydrocephalus, flaccid paraplegia and lack of sphincter control (**96**).

94

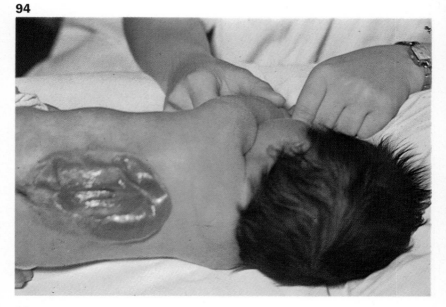

95

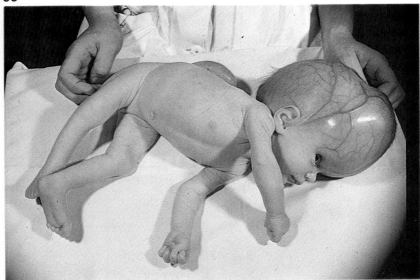

96

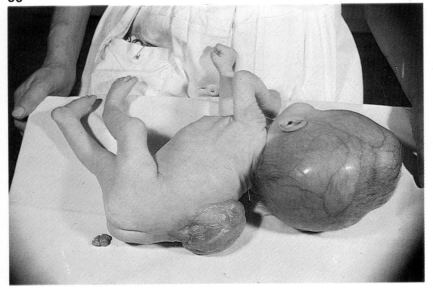

97 Same baby 18 months old. Note the disproportion between the normal size of the face and the grotesque enlargement of the skull. *Visus hydrocephalicus* and engorged scalp veins indicate the increased intra-cranial pressure. At autopsy, the cortex was found to be only paper thin.

98 & 99 Lumbo-sacral myelomeningocele This is the most frequent localisation. There is flexion of the hip joints and knees, paralysis of the feet with talipes equinovarus. The mental capacity was only mildly affected. Operation shortly after birth was refused.

Antenatal detection of neural tube defects and avoidance of recurrence is based on the evaluation of the level of alphafetoprotein (AFP), a foetal globulin, in the maternal serum during the 16th to 18th week of pregnancy.

The correct gestational age can be determined by sonography.

97

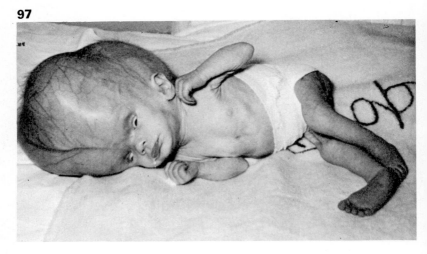

98

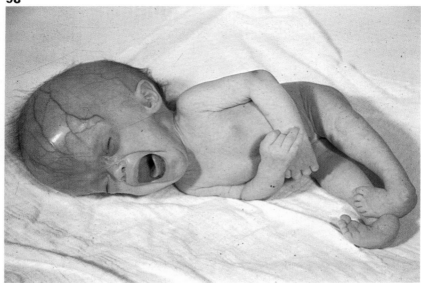

99

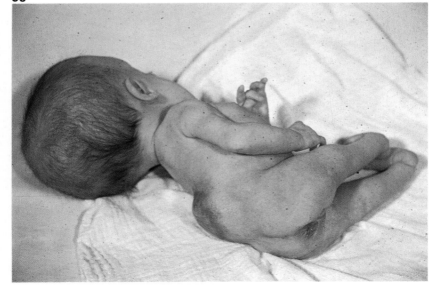

100 Lumbo-sacral teratoma partly covered with normal skin. The tumour contained dental and osseous tissue, hair follicles and viscera. There was no disability after removal.

101 & 102 Anencephaly and hemicrania A severe defect incompatible with survival. Only parts of the posterior skull, brainstem and cerebellum are developed, covered with a vascular membrane (*see cyclopia and arhinencephaly*, **539-541**).

High AFP levels in the maternal serum and in the amniotic fluid are associated with this malformation.

In high risk areas sonography and amniocentesis are indicated within the routine of antenatal care.

100

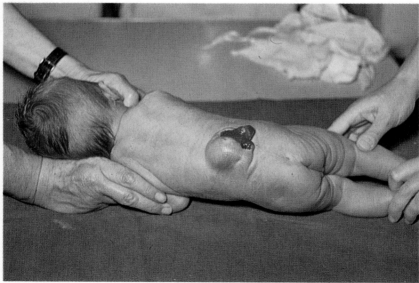

101

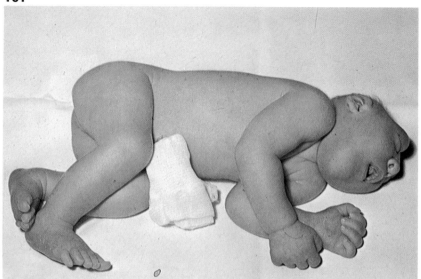

102

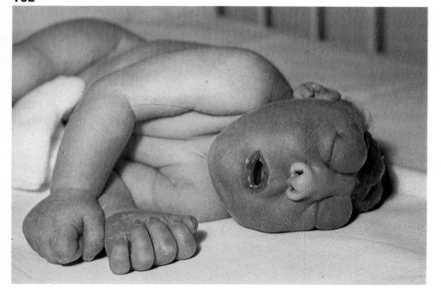

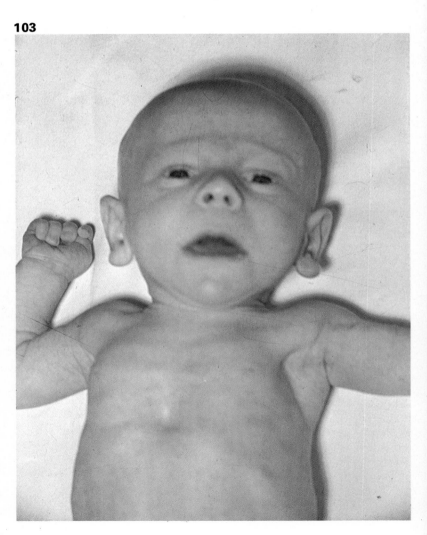

103 Funnel chest Retraction of the lower part of the sternum is due to a short central tendon of the diaphragm and costal deformities.

104 Funnel chest and micrognathia may be associated with respiratory difficulties. Note the right wrist drop (*see* **68, 69**).

104

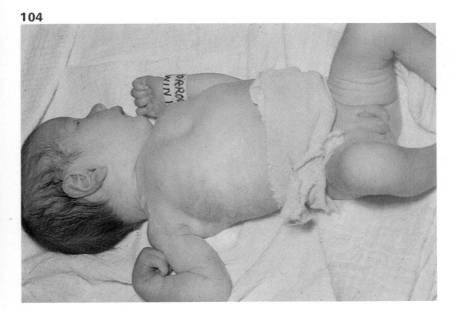

105 Brachydactylia produced by shortness of the metacarpal and phalangeal bones. It appears with various anomalies (*see* **231 & 232**).

106 & 107 Congenital ring constriction (Streeter's dysplasia, pseudo-ainhum) seen around the ankles and toes in a newborn, produced by amniotic bands. The constriction grooves are still visible at 8 years (**107**).

105

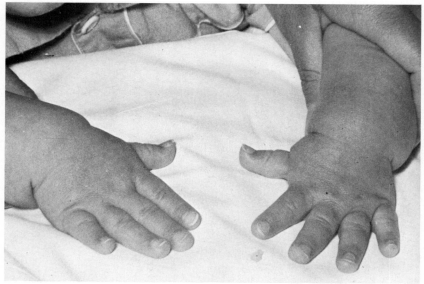

106

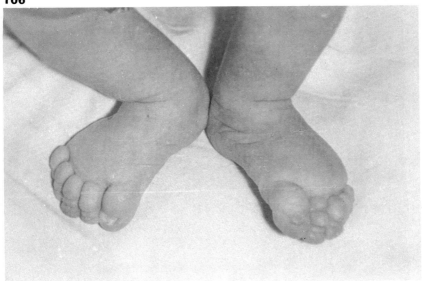

107

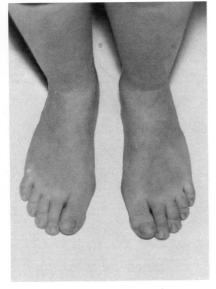

108 Intra-uterine amputation of digits by amniotic strings
following premature rupture of the amniotic sac and oligohydramnios is
a severe degree of the preceding anomaly.

109 Talipes equinovarus A disabling deformity requiring early
correction. Note the bilateral inguinal hernia and hydrocele.

110 Talipes calcaneovalgus A minor deformity with the tendency to
spontaneous improvement.

111 Hemimelia (acromelia) Aplasia of the right fibula. The lower
part of the right leg is hypoplastic ; only the first and second toe are
developed. This deformity has appeared with thalidomide intake among
the most severe forms of multiple bone aplasias.

108

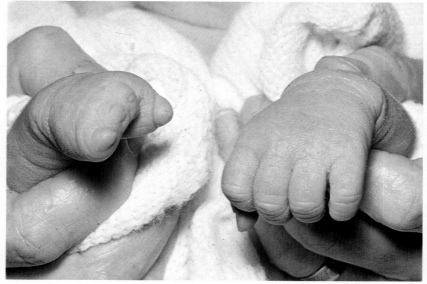

109

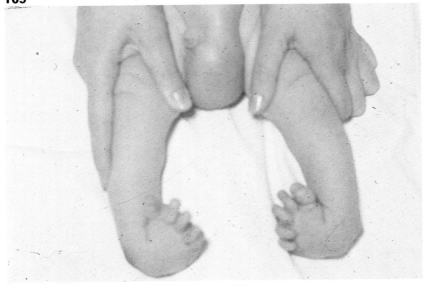

110

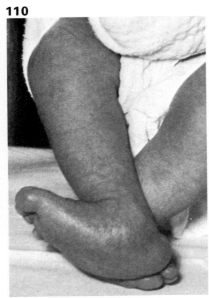

111

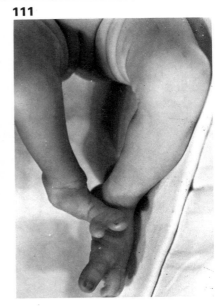

Anomalies of the first embryonic arch can be greatly improved with plastic surgery. It should be done within the first few months for preventive and cosmetic reasons.

112 Unilateral cleft lip (hare lip) extends to the left nostril, which is flattened and deflected.

113 Cleft alveolar ridge and a total cleft of the hard and soft palate is exposed by crying.

114 Cheilo-gnatho-palato-schisis with port-wine-naevus on the affected side. The buccal cavity is covered with monilia.

115 Medianfacial defect shows microcephaly, hypotelorism and a total bilateral cleft. The nasal septum is missing, the nasal and oral cavities are communicating. The deformity is part of holoprosencephaly (*see* **539**).

112

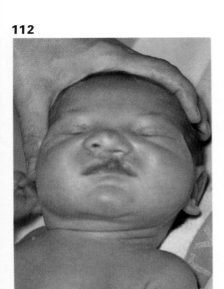

113

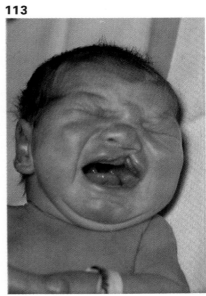

114

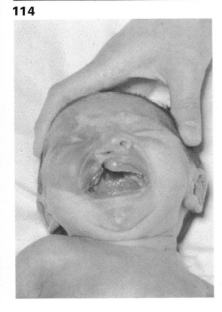

115

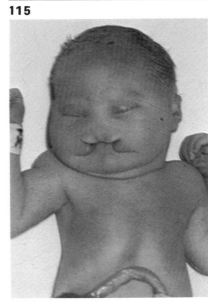

The following cases show the remarkable results of plastic surgery :

116 Unilateral cleft extends into the right nostril. One year after reconstructive surgery (*right*) the appearance has improved considerably.

117 & 118 A severe total cleft with jutting out vomer (117)   One year after operation (**118**) the deformity is hardly noticeable.

116

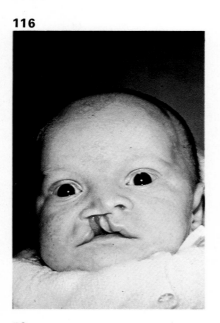 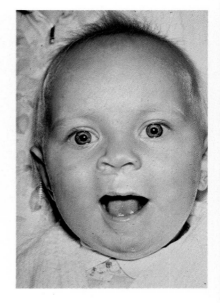

117

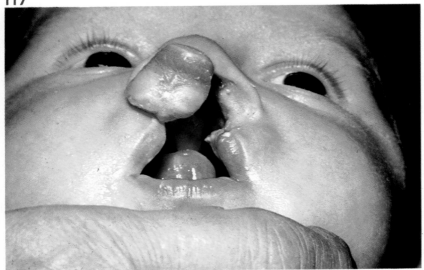

118

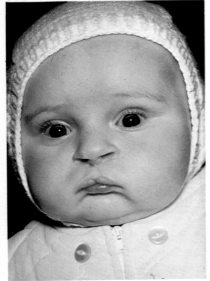

119 Generalised moderate peripheral cyanosis in a shocked new-born with vasomotor instability and poor lung expansion.

120 A 'blue baby' There is severe peripheral and central cyanosis. Post-mortem revealed *Fallot's tetralogy*. Note the malformed low-set ear.

121 & 122 Severe peripheral and central cyanosis Convulsion (**122**) was produced by increased hypoxia after prolonged crying. Post-mortem revealed *atresia of the pulmonary artery* and a *single ventricle*.

119

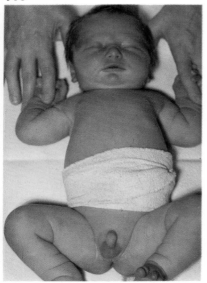

120

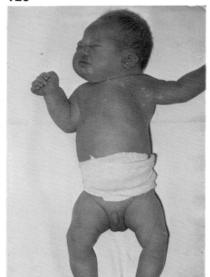

121

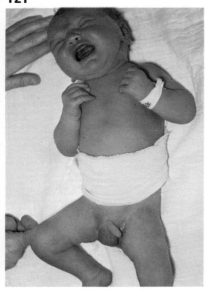

122

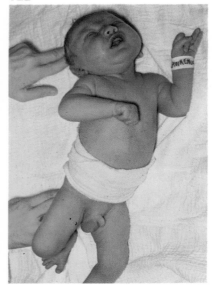

THE UROGENITAL TRACT

123 Neonatal hydrocele Usually transitory ; spontaneous resorption occurs.

124 Bilateral inguinal hernia with large hydrocele Here early correction is indicated.

125 Hypospadias and chordee The urethral orifice is situated ventrally below the glans. Severity varies.

123

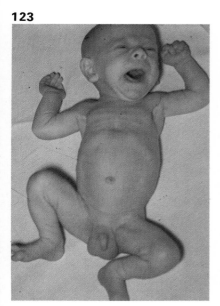

124

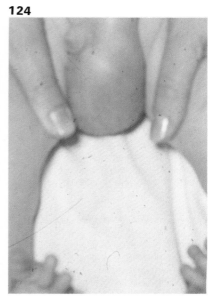

125

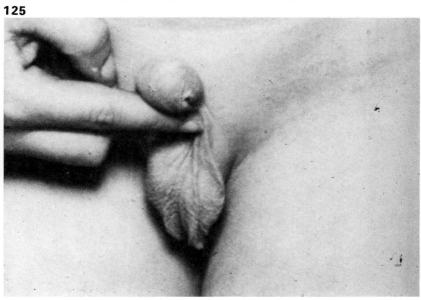

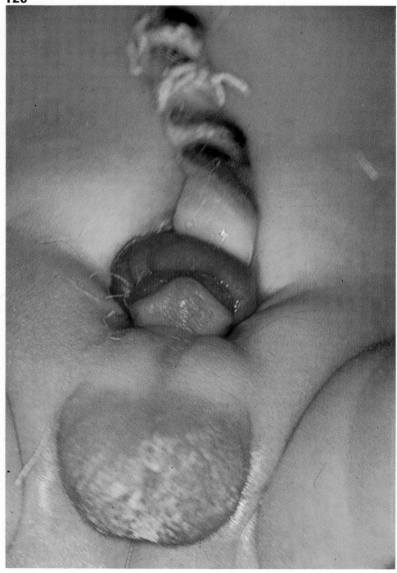

126 Exstrophy of the bladder A developmental arrest which affects males in particular. In the centre below the bright red mucosa of the bladder are the trigonon and the urethral orifices. The short penis shows complete epispadias.

127 Appearance at the age of 11 years The mucosa is replaced by squamous epithelium and scar formation. The exstrophy has shrunk. There is constant dribbling of urine, but the surrounding skin shows little irritation (*see* **566-571** *for other disorders*).

127

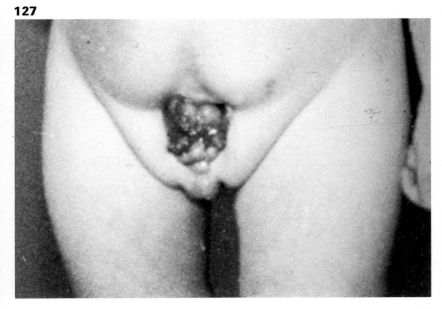

EMERGENCIES

128 Oesophageal atresia with tracheo-oesophageal fistula of the lower segment The baby was vomiting and drooling. The plain x-ray film shows a shadow in the right upper lung and air in the stomach and abdomen.

129 Upper oesophageal segment seen as a dilated blind pouch when outlined by oesophography. The air in the stomach and abdomen indicates communication between trachea and oesophagus. This is the most frequent variety of this malformation.

130 The outline of the bronchial tree due to overflow and aspiration of the contrast fluid. An avoidable incident.

128

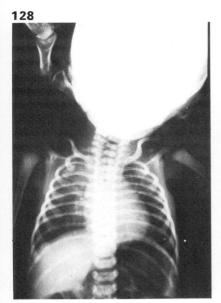

129

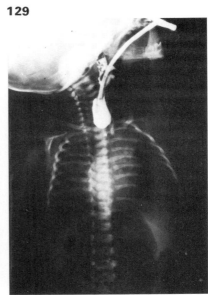

130

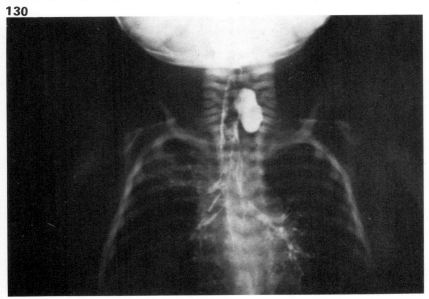

131 Duodenal atresia This baby was a male mongol and vomited bile-stained fluid. The x-ray film taken in supine position outlines the air-filled stomach and duodenum. There is no air elsewhere in the abdomen.

132 Diagnostically significant 'double-bubble' revealed by the x-ray picture taken in upright position.

133 Diaphragmatic hernia through the left pleuroperitoneal canal This 2-day-old baby had respiratory difficulties and repeated cyanotic attacks. The x-ray shows displacement of the heart to the right, and cystic shadows in the left lobe. There is little air in the abdomen.

134 Lateral view presents the airfilled intestinal coils in the thorax.

135 Right-sided diaphragmatic hernia The right lung and mediastinum are shifted to the left. The right diaphragm is depressed, and multiple intestinal coils are in the right thorax. This malformation is less common.

131

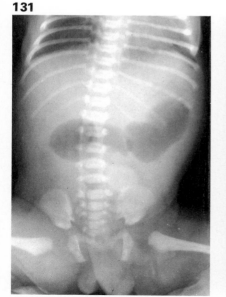

132

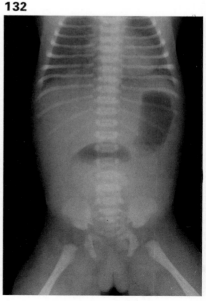

133

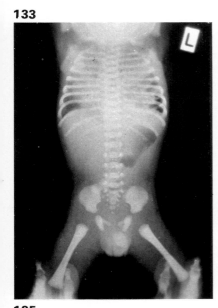

134

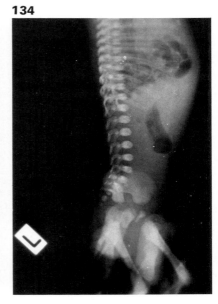

135

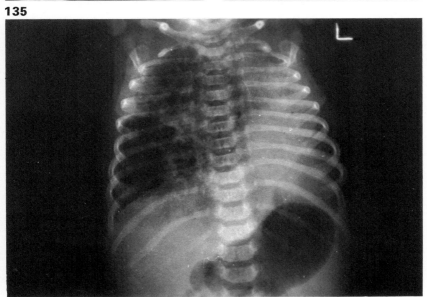

136 Pulmonary unilateral aplasia Post-mortem specimen. New-born with respiratory distress, cyanosis and absence of breath sounds on the right. The heart and mediastinum were shifted to the left by a pleural effusion. Only a small part of the right lung is developed. Less severe defects can be compatible with survival.

137 Exomphalos (omphalocele) A developmental arrest of the abdominal wall around the sixth to eighth foetal week. Rupture of the sac has occurred and there is complete eventration. Immediate surgical correction is imperative (*see* **75-76**).

138 Volvulus and meconium ileus Drawing of a surgical specimen removed from a 6-hour-old infant showing gross dilatation above the twisted part of the lower ileum. The baby later developed *cystic fibrosis of the pancreas* (*see* **275-277**).

136

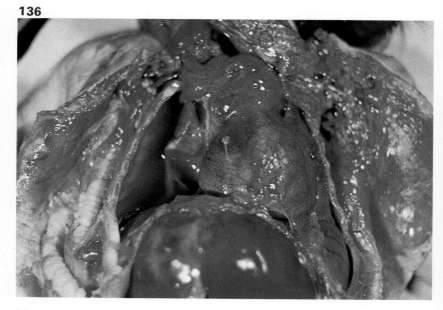

137

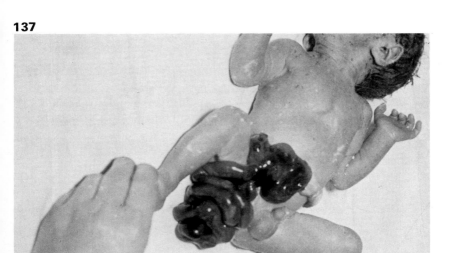

138

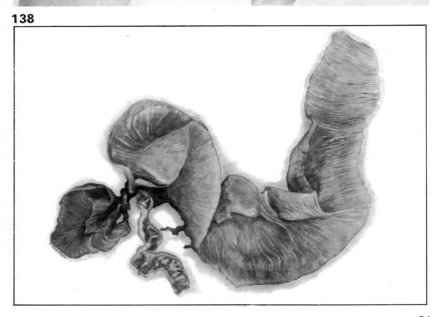

139 Low intestinal obstruction The whole abdomen is distended and there is visible peristalsis.

140 & 141 Diagnostic x-ray pictures In the supine position (**140**) grossly distended intestinal loops can be seen. In the upright position (**141**) after intake of fluid, the significant multiple fluid levels appear.

142 Imperforated anus The anal canal is covered with skin. The baby also had a *cystic kidney* and *hydro-ureter*.

139

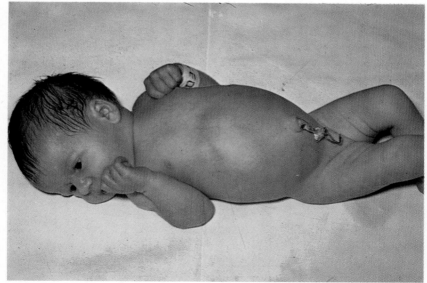

140

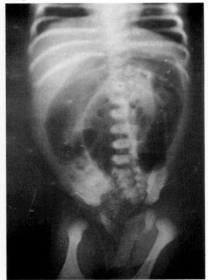

141

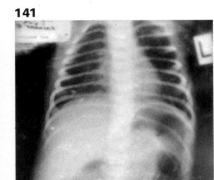

142

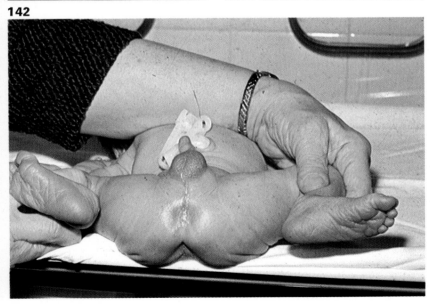

THE INFANT AT RISK

PLACENTAL DYSFUNCTION SYNDROME

143 Macrosomia Oversized babies are either familial or the result of maternal diabetes (*see* **224-228**). Obstetrical and perinatal complications are predominant.

The tendency to overgrowth declines during the first year of life, when normal weight is reached.

Diminished placental permeability and the reduction of intra-uterine oxygen supply produce immediate perinatal difficulties or delayed disability.

144-146 Placental infarction A coloured baby, born at 40 weeks' gestation. The skin is dry, thin and wrinkled. Sparse hair and lack of subcutaneous fat enhance the picture of malnutrition.

143

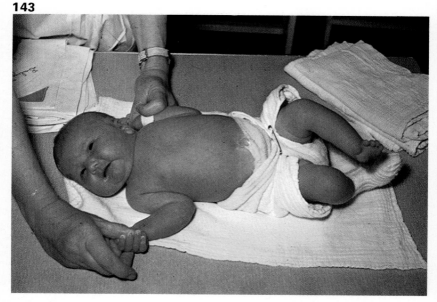

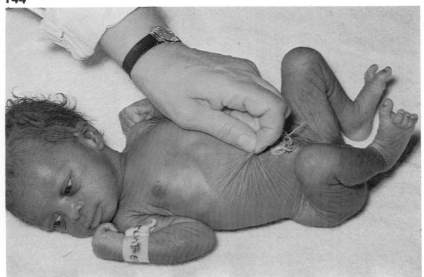

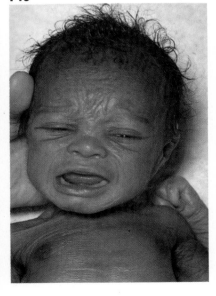

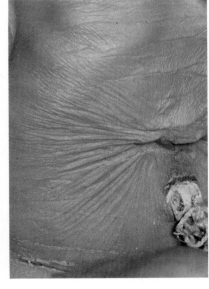

147 & 148 Postmaturity Born at 43 weeks' gestation. Note the peeling, dry skin, scaphoid abdomen and wasted buttocks. The inflammation of the heels is self-inflicted by continuous rubbing.

147

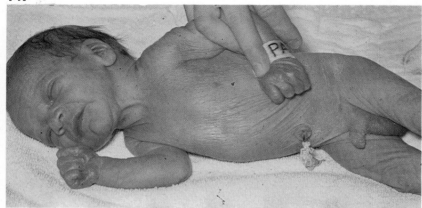

148

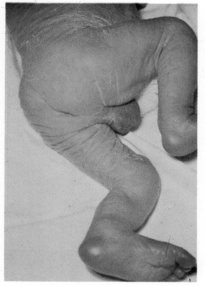

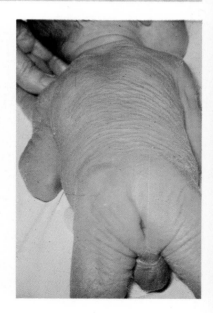

PREMATURITY

Infants born at or below 37 weeks' gestation, with a birthweight below 2500g, run a risk that is proportionate to the causes of prematurity, duration of pregnancy, the birthweight and presence of malformations. The developmental prognosis of prematurity is statistically over-shadowed by the tendency to motor and intellectual disabilities which is more related to the birthweight than to any postnatal complications.

149 General appearance Born at 27 weeks' gestation. Birthweight was 1050g. Note the large head in relation to the body size and the exaggerated foetal flexure posture (*left*). The skin is shiny due to oedema and is covered with lanugo. The subcutaneous fat tissue is poorly developed. The scalp hair is sparse and straight (*right*). The eyes are pro-truding due to disproportion between the size of the eyeballs and the orbital cavity.

149

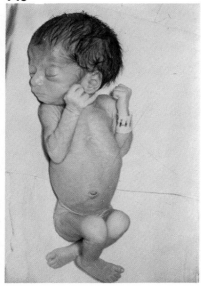 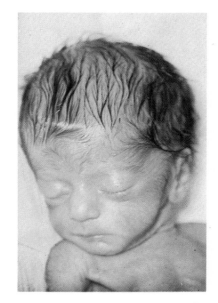

Respiratory distress syndrome, a life-threatening condition associated with complications of pregnancy, labour, prematurity and maternal diabetes, may develop shortly after delivery. Deficient surfactant activity (pulmonary lecithin synthesis) leads to progressive alveolar collapse, hypoxia and metabolic disturbance.

A low lecithin/sphingomyelin ratio (below 2) in the amniotic fluid will predict the risk for the baby.

150 A premature of 28 weeks' gestation Birthweight 1020g. Shows the typical signs of chest retraction, jaundice and cyanosis. Note the glistening gelatinous skin due to oedema.

Assisted ventilation is reducing the high mortality rate. The surviving infants usually show little residual damage.

In threatened premature labour, treatment of the mother with glucocorticoids will reduce the incidence and severity of this syndrome.

151 Wilson-Mikity syndrome Idiopathic, interstitial pneumonitis, a chronic form of respiratory distress. Note the inspiratory retraction of the lower thorax aperture and the bulging abdomen reminiscent of '*seesaw*' breathing. (The chest rises during expiration.)

150

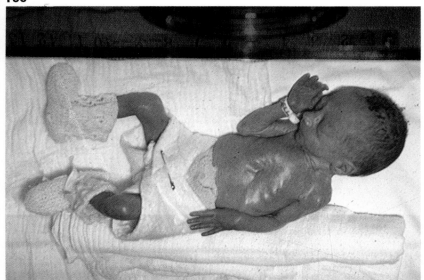

151

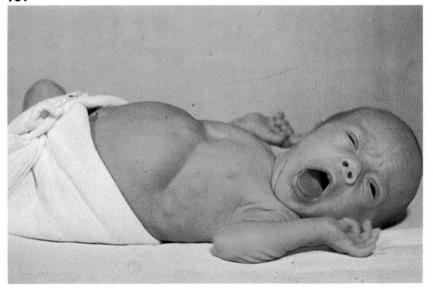

99

Irrespective of possible developmental handicaps, there is a catch-up potential, which justifies the efforts for the survival of these babies.

152 Premature baby of 28 weeks' gestation Birthweight 1021g. Developed respiratory distress of short duration.

153 At 4½ years Height was on the 3rd centile, weight 10th centile, for age. Had recurrent respiratory infections with bronchospasm. Note the retraction of the lower thoracic cage (*Harrison sulcus*) and abdominal distension (*top, right*). **At 11 years** (*bottom*) she was a well-grown, healthy, pubertal girl. Thelarche (*incipient breast development*) is visible. Height on 25th centile, weight 50th centile. IQ 110. The respiratory attacks have ceased.

152

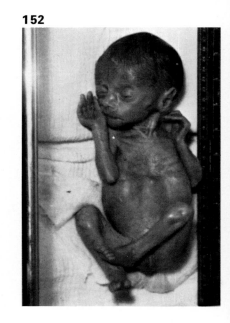

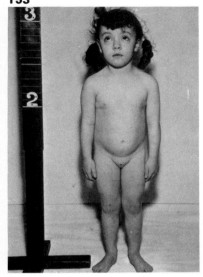
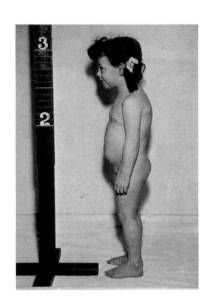
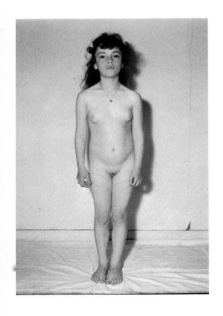
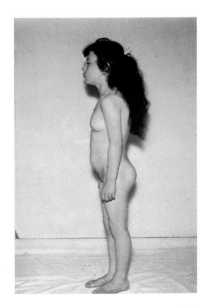

MULTIPLE PREGNANCY

The perinatal risk of prematurity and low birthweight is intensified by the inborn complications of twinning and obstetric difficulties. Twin pregnancies are relatively frequent (*1:80 pregnancies*). Non-identical (*fraternal*) dizygous twins are more common than identical monozygous ones. Some of the problems associated with twinning are shown.

154 Identical twins born by Caesarian section at 37 weeks. The mother had diabetes. Both babies show oedema and relative macrosomia (*see* **38, 143**).

155 Non-identical sex-like twins, breech and forceps delivery at 39 weeks. Both babies are small-for-date. The second (*forceps*) twin was cyanotic and had to be resuscitated.

Intra-uterine growth retardation (birthweight below the 10th centile for gestational age) predisposes increased perinatal mortality, especially in twin pregnancy. Control of the biparietal growth of the foetal head by ultrasound may be predictive.

156 Dizygous twins of different sex not identified during pregnancy. Normal delivery at 42 weeks. Both babies are mature and well-developed.

154

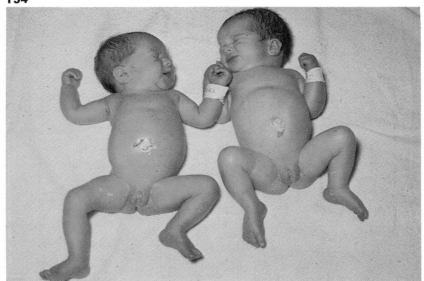

155

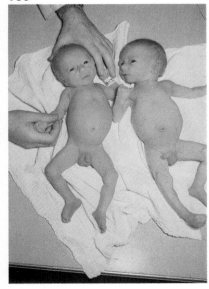

156

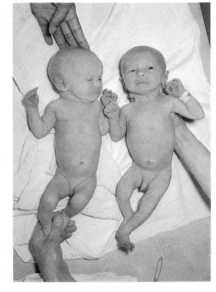

157 Dizygous sex-like twins born at 36 weeks' gestation. Birth-weight differed by 1kg. The placenta of the second twin was small. This baby developed respiratory distress.

158 Intra-uterine transfusion syndrome after foetus-to-foetus transfusion via an arteriovenous shunt in monozygous monochorionic twins. The donor is smaller and mildly anaemic, the recipient is hyper-volaemic.

159 The same syndrome in a severer form Note the marked anaemia and dystrophy of the donor and the serious plethora of the recipient at birth. This baby had to be relieved by withdrawal of blood and the anaemic twin had to be transfused.

157

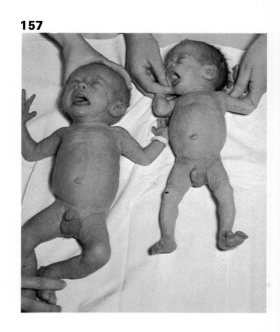

158

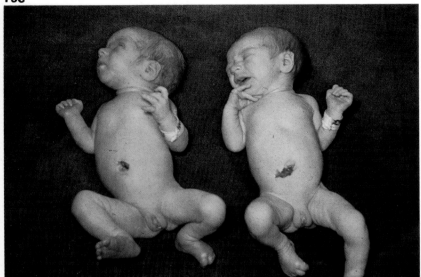

159

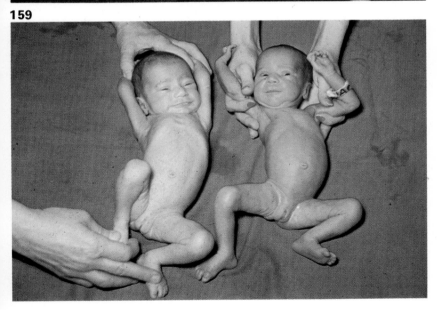

DISEASES OF THE NEWBORN

BACTERIAL INFECTIONS

160 Neonatal tetanus in a West African baby. Infection occurred via the umbilical wound. The child is seen in a convulsion with neck retraction and extensor spasm of the crossed limbs. The severe trismus is producing feeding difficulties.

161 Umbilical septicaemia Note the severe dystrophy and abdominal distention. Post-mortem revealed inflammation of the umbilical and hypogastric vessels, liver abscesses and peritonitis. *Bacterium Escherich coli* was isolated.

162 Neonatal meningitis The bulging anterior fontanelle indicates cerebral oedema and incipient hydrocephalus. *Staphylococcus pyogenes* was cultured from the cerebrospinal fluid.

160

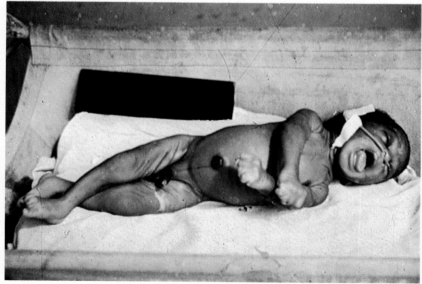

161

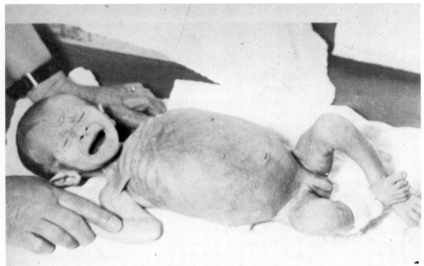

162

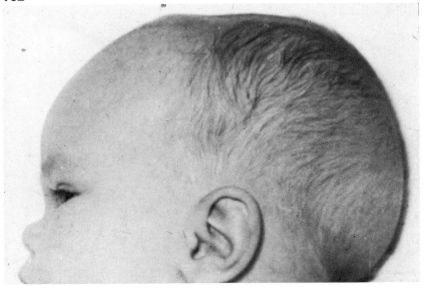

163 Incipient pyodermia The vesicle surrounded by an inflammatory halo (*arrowed*) contained coagulase-positive *Staphylococcus pyogenes*. A highly infectious condition requiring strict isolation.

164 & 165 Dermatitis exfoliativa (the scalded skin syndrome, Ritter's disease) in a 7-week-old infant. Superficial blisters and erosions have formed and the skin peels off over wide areas on touching (*Nikolsky phenomenon*).

Antibiotics and steroids have dramatically improved the prognosis of this pyogenic condition.

163

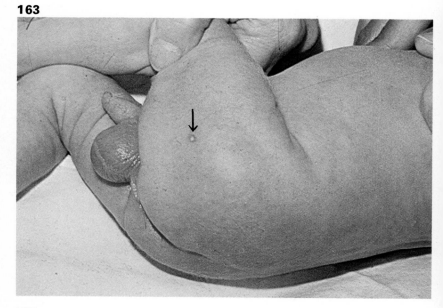

164

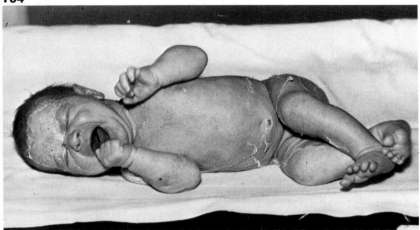

165

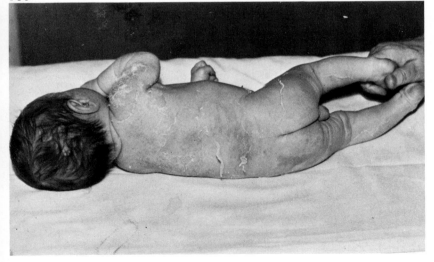

166 Haemorrhagic stomatitis The mother had scarlet fever.
β-haemolytic streptococcus group A was isolated.

**167-169 Disseminated intravascular coagulation syndrome
(consumption coagulopathy, defibrination syndrome)** An
acquired disorder of haemostasis concurrent with other conditions
leading to thrombosis, widespread haemorrhage and necrosis. This
premature baby of 30 weeks' gestation has oedema and haemorrhage
of the penis and phalangeal joints, and a generalised toxic erythema
(*see* **75**).

166

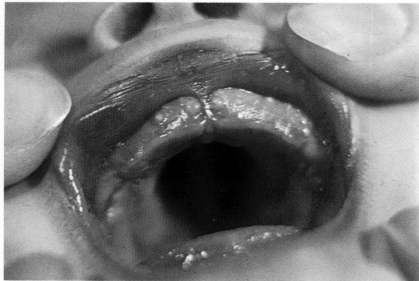

167

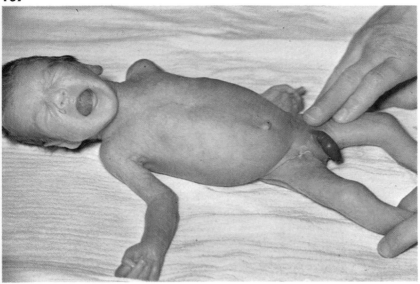

168

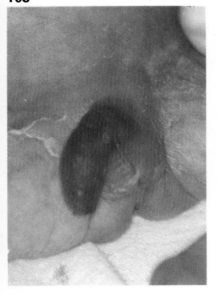

169

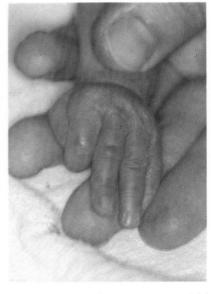

170 Purpura fulminans (Sanarelli-Schwartz phenomenon) The severest degree of this syndrome in a premature of 28 weeks' gestation. Note the grey colour of the body, the intense purpuric acrocyanosis of hands and feet with incipient necrosis.

Bacterial or viral infections are usually preceding. High doses of corticosteroids together with fibrinogen, and fresh plasma infusion may arrest progression.

170

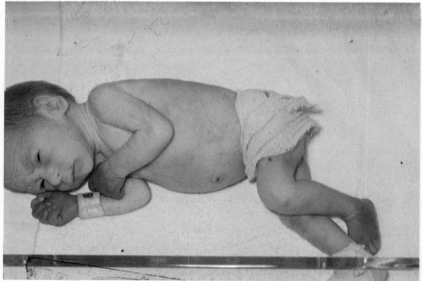

FUNGAL INFECTIONS

(Occur more frequently in bottle fed infants)

171 Oral monilia (thrush) An infection with *Candida albicans* common in the neonate, usually transmitted by maternal infection. The white plaques on the tongue and buccal cavity resemble milk curds, but cannot be removed easily. One twin only was affected which indicates an individual susceptibility to the infection.

172 Skin thrush Note the characteristic epithelial fringe around the follicles and vesicles on an otherwise normal skin.

171

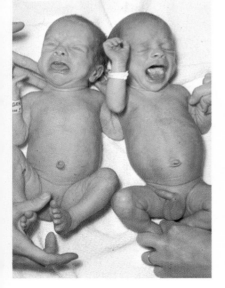

172

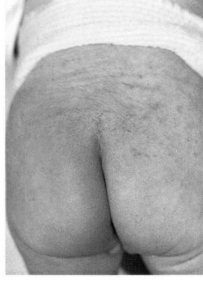

173 Weeping dermatitis in the genito-crural area superinfected with monilia. The backview shows the rash confined to the area of napkin/diaper contact.

174 & 175 Disseminated moniliasis Note the confluent erythema of the scalp, face and genito-crural area. The body is covered with isolated psoriasiform plaques. Pulmonary infection occurs by aspiration. The backview (**175**) shows mainly erythema and some isolated plaques in the gluteal area.

173

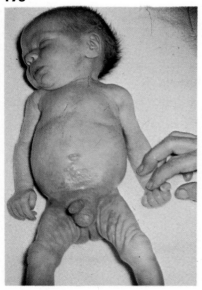
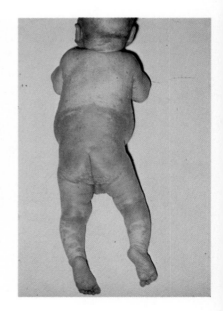

174

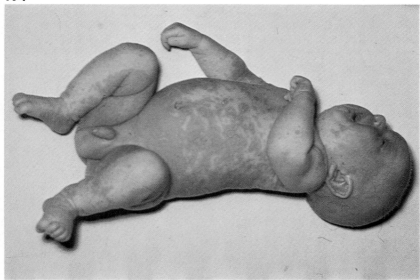

175

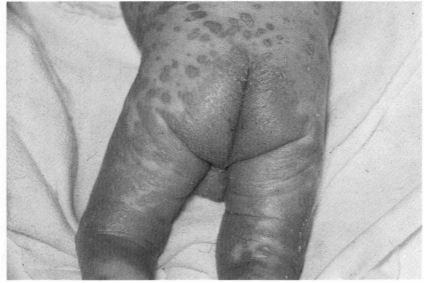

176 & 177 Dermatitis seborrhoides (Moro) appears within the first trimester, and is more frequent in breastfed infants. Biotin deficiency of breastmilk is postulated. The face, neck, axillary folds and the genito-crural area are mainly affected. In contrast to *eczema*, the scalp and the extremities remain free.

178 & 179 Sensitivity reaction to local therapy Treatment consisted of a lotion containing neomycin and zinc oxide. The white cradle cap is talcum powder.

176

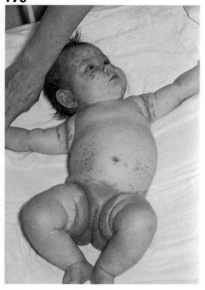
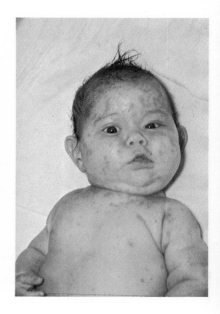

177

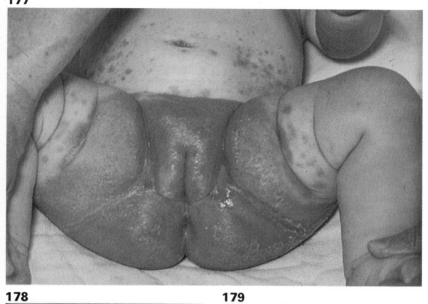

178

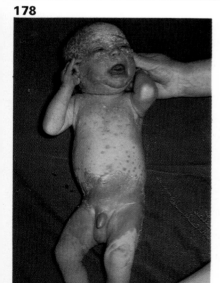

179

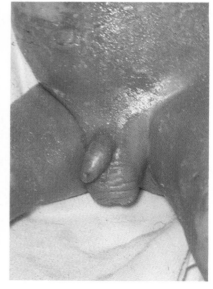

180-182 The healing stage Note the residual seborrhoea on the forehead, eyebrows and lids (**180**). On the abdomen and buttocks (**181**) the rash resolves in psoriasiform patches ; in the genito-crural area (**182**) the skin is dry and indurated. There is usually no recurrence.

180

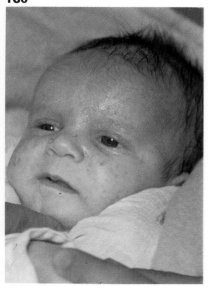

181

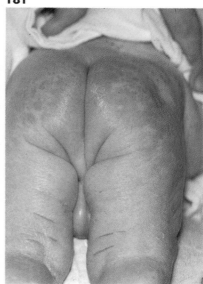

182

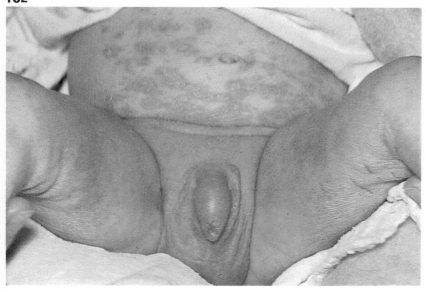

119

183 Erythrodermia desquamativa (Leiner's disease) A dyskeratosis. Coarse, greasy, 'potato-chip'-like scales cover principally the face and trunk. Failure to thrive, eosinophilia and diarrhoea are additional features. Protein deficiency of the diet, especially with breast feeding, was considered in the aetiology. Dietary adjustment and local application of steroids are effective.

184 & 185 Napkin/diaper psoriasis (Psoriasoid Jadassohn-Tachau) Erythema, lichenification and peeling are confined to the napkin/diaper area. The disorder is difficult to treat and prone to relapse.

183

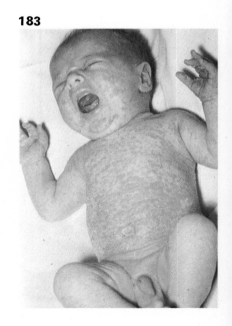

184

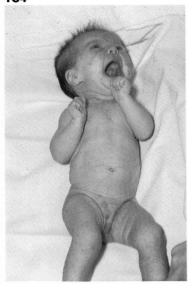
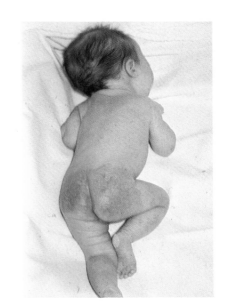

185

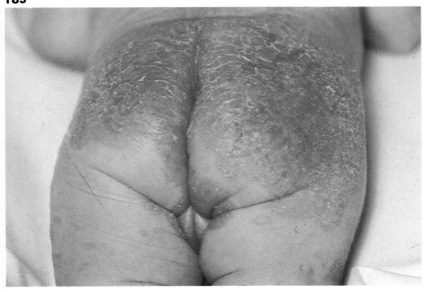

Lamellar ichthyosis (collodion baby) (186-193) A disturbance of keratinisation of autosomal, recessive inheritance.

The condition has to be differentiated from the 'Harlequin Baby', the severest form of congenital ichthyosis, where shedding of the thick keratinous membrane does not occur. Affected infants do not survive.

186-189 Appearance at birth The baby is encased in a collodion-like skin, the face, eyes and ears are distorted, the fingers and toes compressed and oedematous.

186

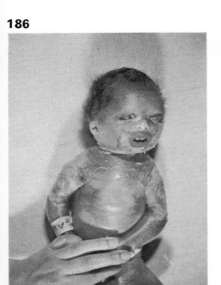

187

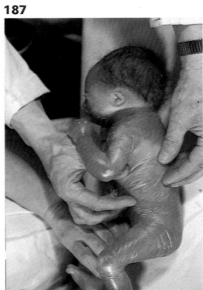

188

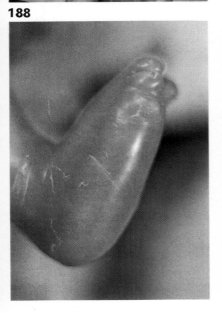

189

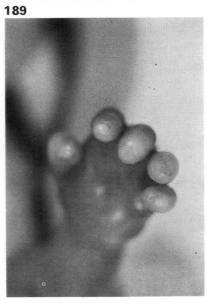

190 One week later cracks and lamellar desquamation formed. The superficial membrane has peeled off exposing a softer skin. The compressed parts are unfolding.

191 At 3 weeks the skin is now smooth, bright red and glistening. The features are normal.

192 & 193 At 18 months A well-developed child. The skin is thick, scaly and itching. The nails are dystrophic. This state is permanent.

190

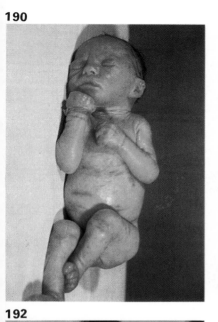

191

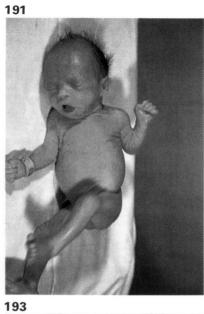

192

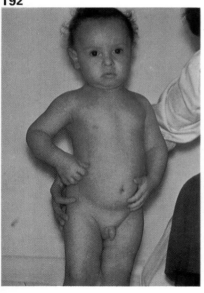

193

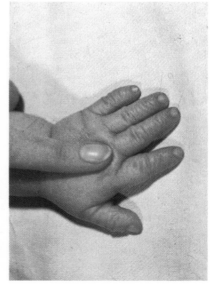

BLOOD DISORDERS

194 Congenital thrombocytopenic purpura This Indian baby developed generalised purpura, thrombocytopenia and prolonged bleeding time. Mother's serum contained platelet antibodies. This condition can occur with intra-uterine rubella infection and congenital syphilis. The cushingoid appearance is the result of steroid treatment.

195 Erythrocytosis, neonatal polycythaemia An adaptation to prolonged hypoxia. Compare the colour of the affected premature of 34 weeks' gestation with that of the unaffected infant. Pathologic polycythaemia has to be excluded.

Intra-uterine growth retardation may be contributory. Relief of the polycythaemia and hyperviscosity may be necessary (*see* **158** *and* **159**).

194

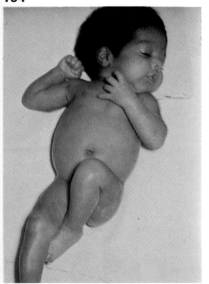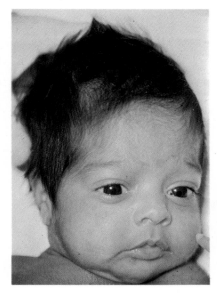

195

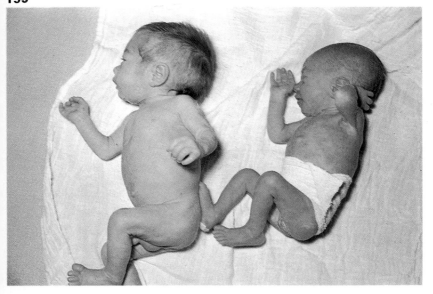

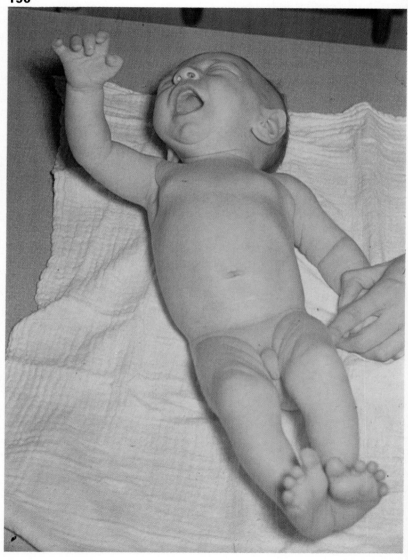

196 Congenital anaemia due to foetal-maternal transfusion. Foetal erythrocytes and haemoglobin appear in mother's blood after delivery.

197 Haemorrhagic disease of the newborn A transitory pro-thrombin, vitamin K and coagulation factor VII deficiency, more frequent in coloured infants. The newborn has *melaena* and *vaginal bleeding*. Administration of water-soluble vitamin K analogue at birth has become a routine preventive procedure.

197

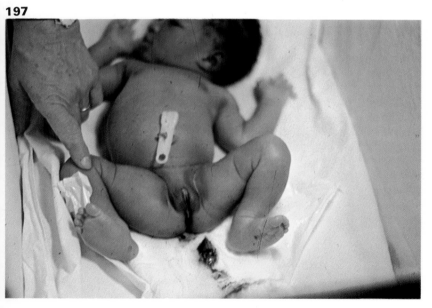

HAEMOLYTIC DISEASE OF THE NEWBORN

The following five pictures illustrate haemolytic disease of the newborn due to maternal izo-immunization during pregnancy. The antigenic difference between maternal and foetal erythrocytes in the Rh or ABO system leads to the destruction of the latter by maternal antibodies. The severity of the manifestation varies.

Prenatal analysis of the amniotic fluid by amniocentesis and amnioscopy has considerably advanced the therapeutic approach.

198 Haemolytic anaemia is the mildest form, liable to spontaneous recovery. The jaundice is moderate.

199 Icterus gravis Hyperbilirubinaemia exceeding the serum level of 20mg/100ml is liable to produce *kernicterus* by uptake of bilirubin into basal ganglia cells. Compared with the physiological jaundice in a premature (*left*) the intensity of the jaundice is obvious. Measures to reduce the serum bilirubin level are imperative.

200 The picture of kernicterus Note the neck-retraction, the hypertonic extensor spasm of the limbs and the intense jaundice. Severe motor and intellectual disability results.

198

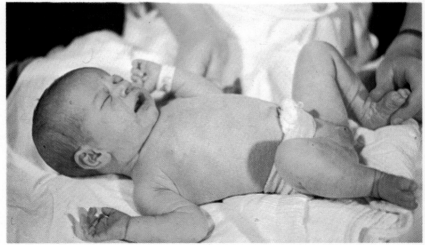

199

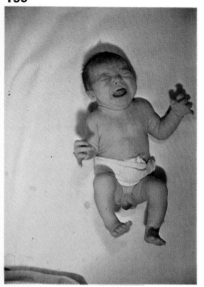

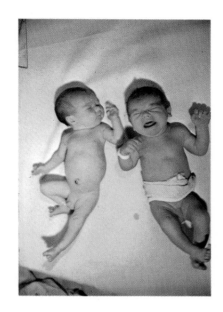

200

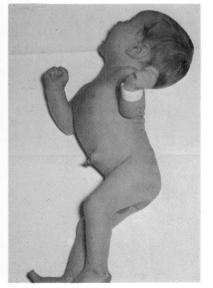

201 Erythroblastosis foetalis The most severe manifestation. A macerated stillborn with *hydrops foetalis*, ascites, hepatosplenomegaly and high-grade anaemia.

202 The placenta shows oedema and infarction on the maternal side (*left*) and pallor on the foetal surface (*right*). The cord is haemorrhagic and oedematous.

In severely affected babies intra-uterine transfusion antenatally of compatible erythrocytes and exchange transfusion postnatally is often lifesaving and effective for the correction of anaemia and the prevention of neurotoxisity from hyperbilirubinaemia.

Injection of anti-D immunoglobulin within a few hours after delivery will reduce the initial sensitisation of Rh negative mothers and the incidence of the disease. The injection of anti-D at 28 and 34 weeks of gestation can also reduce sensitisation during the first pregnancy.

201

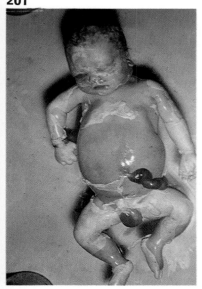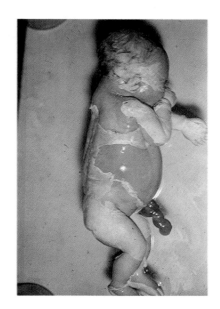

202

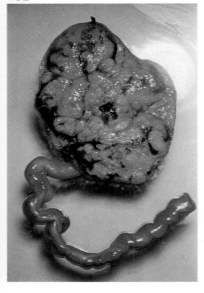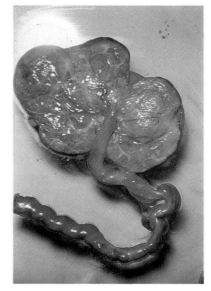

JAUNDICE

203 Physiological jaundice An unconjugated transitory hyperbilirubinaemia appearing within the 2nd and the 6th day after birth due to deficient enzyme glucuronyl-transferase activity and immaturity of liver function to metabolise bilirubin.

204 Breastmilk jaundice A prolonged, benign, unconjugated hyperbilirubinaemia in breastfed babies, due to inhibition of conjugation by a steroid (3-α, 20-β *pregnanediol*) excreted in breastmilk in some cases.

205 Infective hepatitis A conjugated hyperbilirubinaemia due to biliary obstruction by *cholangitis*. Note abdominal distension due to hepatomegaly.

206 Inspissated bile syndrome following meconium ileus, relieved by colostomy. The infant later developed *cystic fibrosis of the pancreas* (*see* **138, 275-277**).

203

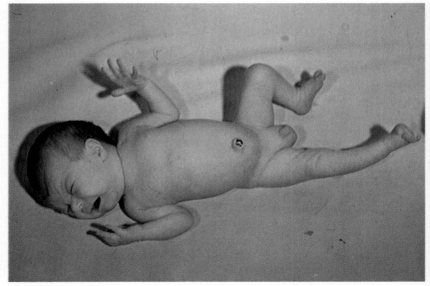

204

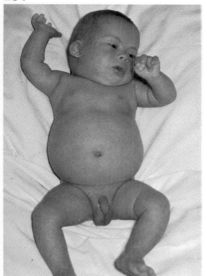

205

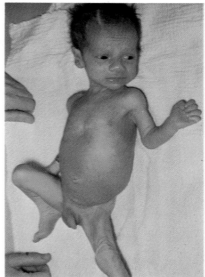

206

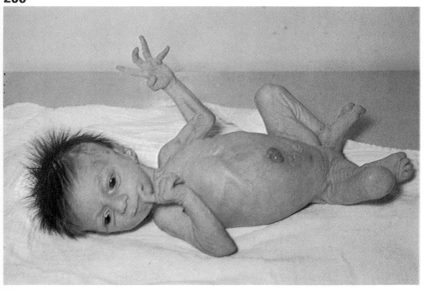

Biliary atresia (207-213) The meconium was acholic (*see* **632**) and jaundice developed shortly after delivery. Parents refused operation.

207 Appearance at 3 months Jaundice is moderate and the nutritional condition is fair. The abdomen is distended, the liver enlarged.

208 At 6 months there is marked dystrophy, pallor and ascites.

209 At 17 months further deterioration. Note the severe emaciation and large abdomen due to *ascites*.

207

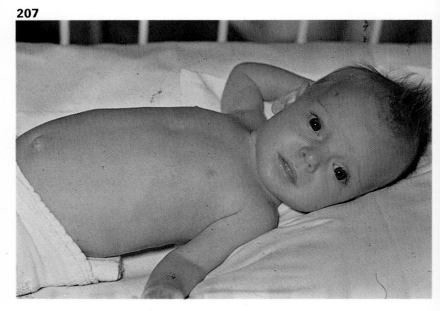

208

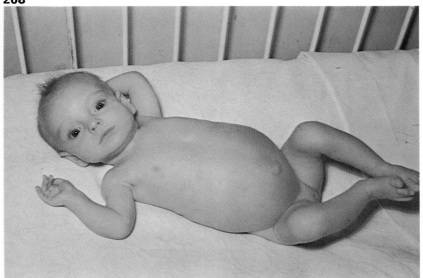

209

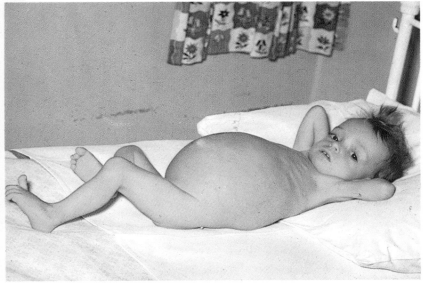

210-212 Additional signs There is scleral jaundice and a greenish colour of the teeth (**210**). Clubbing of fingers and toes (**211 & 212**) has developed.

Surgical correction of extrahepatic obstruction before the 12th week of age is successful. In intrahepatic biliary atresia, where prolonged survival is possible, the treatment is symptomatic.

210

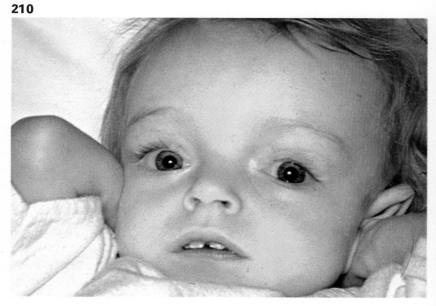

211

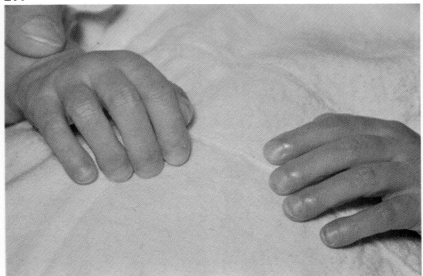

212

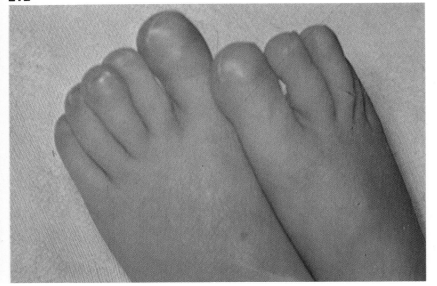

213 At 2 years Note the dark green discoloration of the skin and the grossly distended abdomen. Exploratory laparatomy revealed *biliary cirrhosis* and *intra-* and *extrahepatic aplasia of the bile ducts*. The baby died shortly afterwards.

213

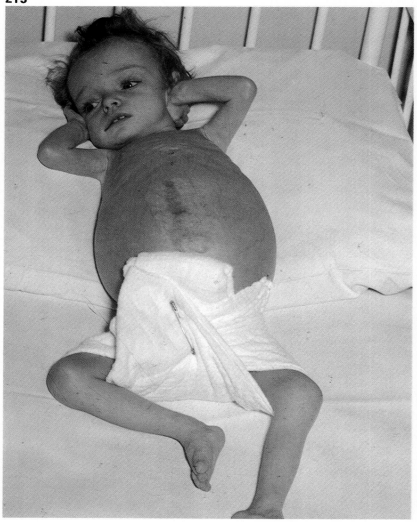

EFFECT OF MATERNAL HORMONES AND DISEASES

The physiological transplacental exchange of hormones between mother and child has been firmly established. The discovery by Norman Gregg in 1941 of the teratogenic potential of *maternal rubella infection* during the early months of pregnancy, and more recently the *thalidomide tragedy*, has alerted attention to the hazards of diseases and medication during pregnancy. Avoidance of known or potential teratogenic interactions and, if necessary, prenatal diagnosis by amniocentesis and amnioscopy, and selective abortion have become indicative.

214 & 215 Neonatal facial acne Appears within the first trimester; a common, transitory, self-limiting disorder produced by maternal androgens. This should not be mistaken for an infective condition.

216 Skin pigmentation resembles maternal pigment changes of the vulva, inner aspect of thighs and the areola. Note the *linea nigra (pregnancy line)* on the abdomen and the *neonatal leukorrhoea.* The latter is a response to maternal hormone withdrawal.

217 & 218 Pigmentation is more marked in coloured infants

214

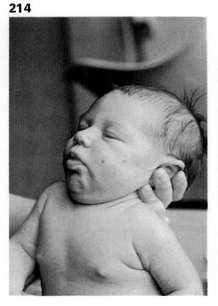

215

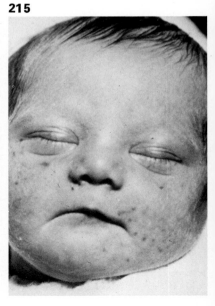

216

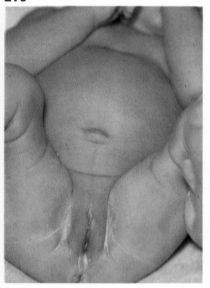

217

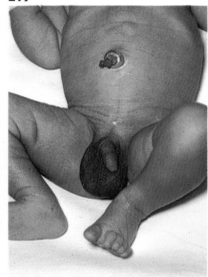

218

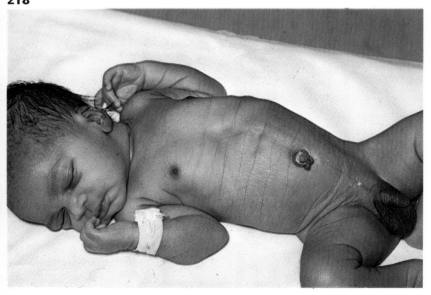

219 Neonatal breast infiltration accompanied by temporary lactation of *witch's milk* (chemically identical with colostrum), a response to maternal hormones.

220 Neonatal mastitis A pyogenic infection, liable to follow expression of the infiltrated breast ; may lead to suppuration and scarring.

221 Neonatal hyperthyroidism induced by LATS (long-acting thyroid stimulator) transferred from the mother, who had been suffering from active Graves' disease. Note the exophthalmos and the dystrophy in the hyperactive baby. The condition is self-limiting, but antithyroid treatment may be necessary initially (*see* **405**).

222 Moderate exophthalmos seen in baby's brother born one year later.

219

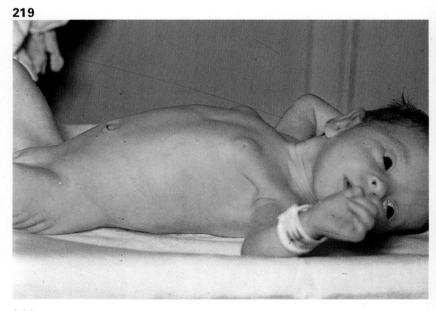

220

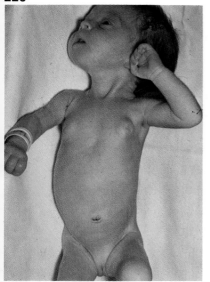

221

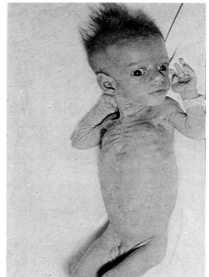

222

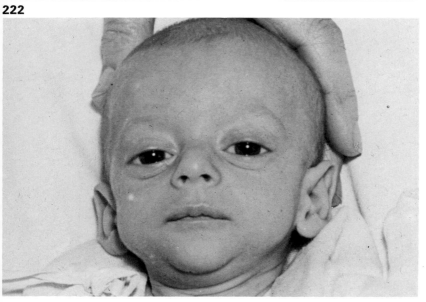

223 Transitory myxoedema in a baby of 2 weeks (*left*). During pregnancy the mother had been treated with goitrogenic drugs. Three months later (*right*) the same baby shows startling recovery (*see 393 & 394*).

Infants of diabetic mothers (224-228) run a high risk of antenatal, obstetric and perinatal complications. Some characteristic features are illustrated.

224 Macrosomia and plethora are the result of intra-uterine over-nutrition and hyperplasia of the adipose tissue (*see 143*).

225 Cushingoid appearance with *balloon cheeks* and plethora. Cortisone serum levels were normal.

223

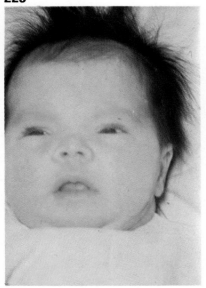
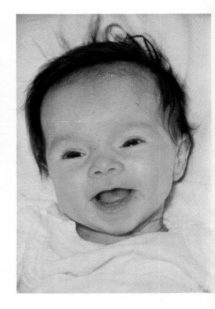

224

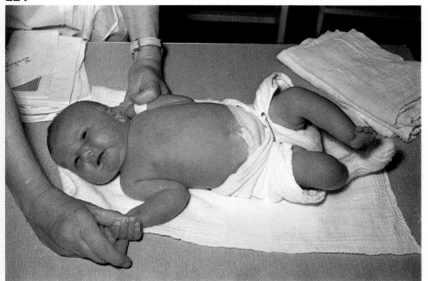

225

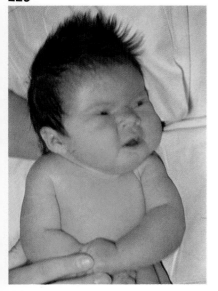

226 Another case Microcephaly, pitting oedema of the limbs, flexion contractures of fingers and toes (*partial arthrogryposis*) and vascular naevi on chest and legs.

227 & 228 Appearance at the age of 1 year Note the marked microcephaly, squint and persistent arthrogryposis. Later the infant developed a severe spastic tetraplegia.

226

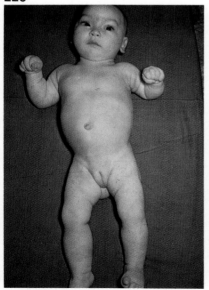

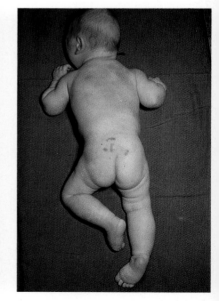

227

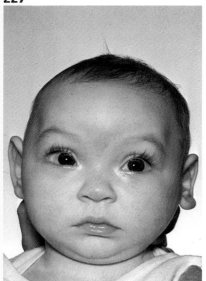

228

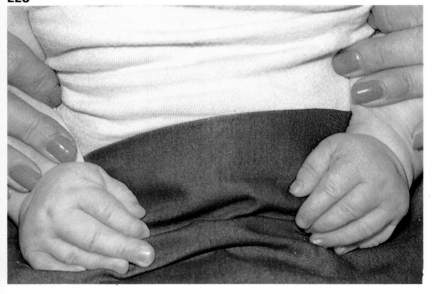

229 & 230 Rubella syndrome Consisting in this case of unilateral cataract and blepharo-spasm. A congenital heart defect was also found. The infant remained retarded. Infection of the mother occurred at five weeks' pregnancy.

231 & 232 A similar case At 17 months, the child had left-sided cataract, microphthalmia and brachydactylia. Height was below the 3rd centile. At the age of 9 years the bone age was only 3.7 years. She remained retarded and dwarfed.

At family planning, mother's immunity to rubella should be ascertained. If susceptible to infection active immunisation is indicated (*see* **357**).

Contact with rubella by susceptible mothers within the first three months of pregnancy carries a high risk of congenital malformation.

229

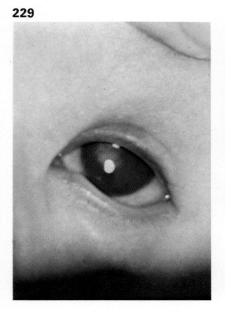

230

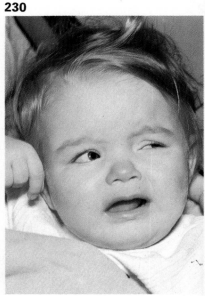

231

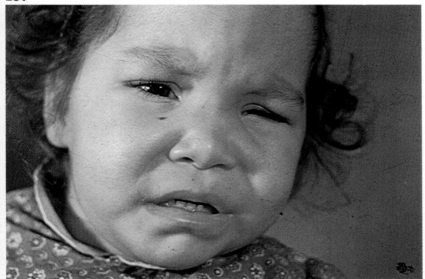

232

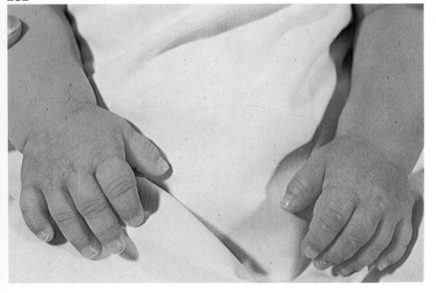

233 & 234 Non-adrenal virilisation (pseudo-hermaphroditism)
A female chromatin-positive infant. The mother had received methyltestosterone in early pregnancy. There is partial fusion of the labia majora
and enlargement of the clitoris resembling hypospadias (*see* **411 & 412**).

233

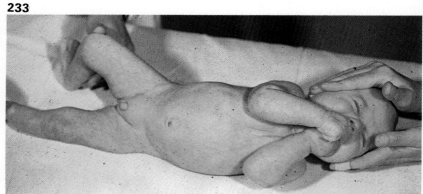

234

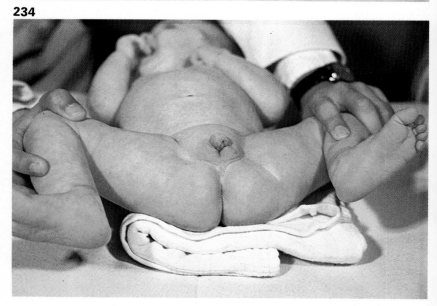

Infancy and Childhood

The pattern of diseases in this age group has been changing. Preventive measures have considerably reduced the incidence of infectious diseases and advances in therapy have improved the prognosis of many other diseases.

Significant results of biochemical research could identify formerly obscure conditions leading to progressive physical and mental decline, such as inborn errors of metabolism, based on particular enzyme defects, detectable by screening in the neonatal period. In consequence, resigned acceptance has been turned into promising therapeutic activity.

The spectacular breakthrough by cytogenetics has illuminated the gloomy pathway of inherited disorders and made it possible to calculate the recurrence risk. Genetic counselling will allow appropriate family planning where adverse predispositions exist.

However, there still remains a wide range of disorders affecting the child's development and adjustment which demand the intensification and reorganisation of medical and social care on a communal scale.

A number of conditions likely to be encountered between infancy and puberty have been selected for presentation in this chapter.

DEVELOPMENTAL MILESTONES

Simultaneously with intellectual and emotional maturation, muscular
activity gradually changes from the involuntary reflex response of the
newborn to voluntary co-ordinate movements performed with increasing
skill.

Undue delay in the sequence requires exploration of the retarding
causes.

235 At 6-8 weeks Head and neck control in prone position.

236 At 3 months Able to raise head and chest.

237 & 238 At 4 months Limbs are now stretched, stands with support.

235

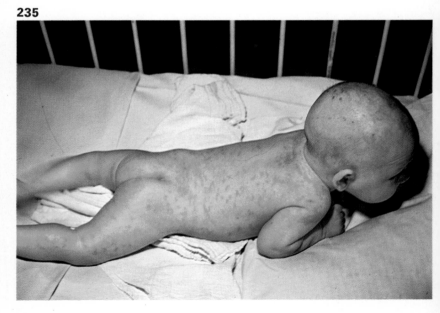

236

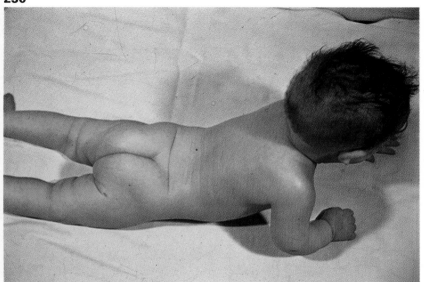

237

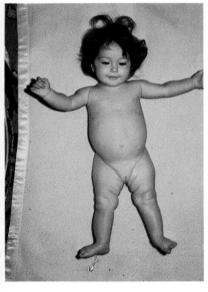

238

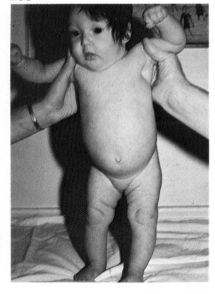

239 At 5 months Sitting with support. Note the sitting kyphosis.

240 & 241 At 8 months Sitting without support, but sitting kyphosis is still retained.

242 At 8-10 months Standing.

243 At 10-12 months Crawling.

239

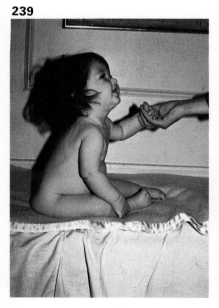

240

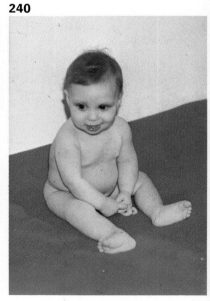

241

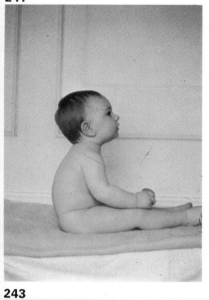

242

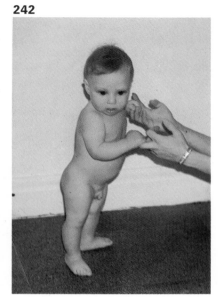

243

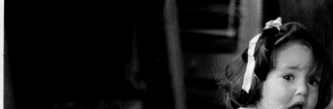

244 At 12-14 months First steps.

245 At 16 months Postural control and co-ordinate hand and finger movements. Note the knock knees and broad base stance.

246 At 3-4 years Fully controlled posture.

244

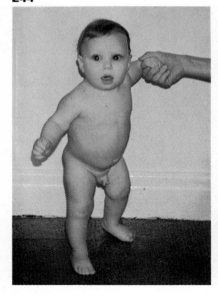

245

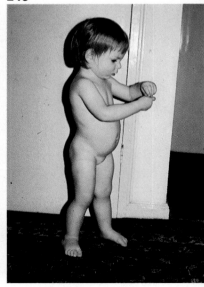

246

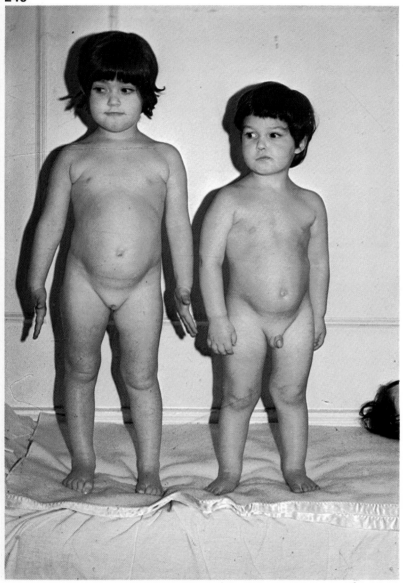

VARIANTS

247 Hypothyroid infant aged 4 months, has poor head and neck control.

248 Same infant at 6 months Foetal flexure of limbs and abduction of the hip joint are still maintained.

249 Hydrocephalus 17-month-old, sitting with support. Lack of head and neck control because of the overweight head.

250 Brain-damaged child 18-month-old, showing severe opisthotonus and exaggerated flexure posture.

247

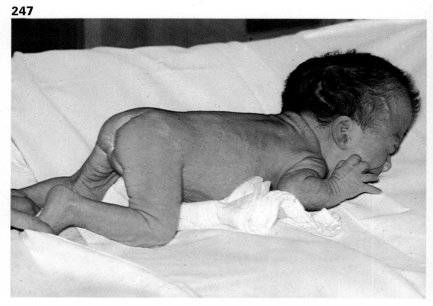

248

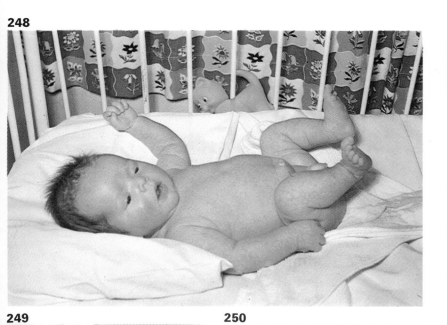

249

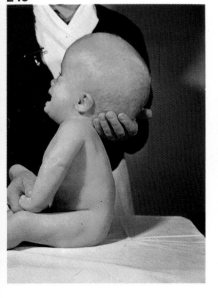

250

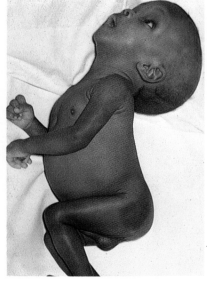

251 Congenital cyanotic heart disease in a 3-year-old. The *Buddha posture* is a variant of squatting.

252 Lumbosacral lordosis in a 3-year-old is compensatory to abdominal distension.

253 Down's syndrome At $2\frac{1}{2}$ years, shows considerable lack of balance due to muscular hypotony. To compensate the girl stands with legs apart and knees over-extended.

251

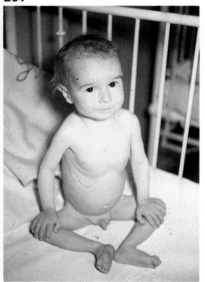

252

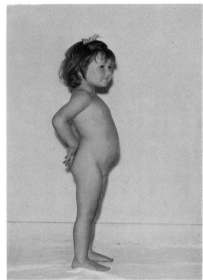

253

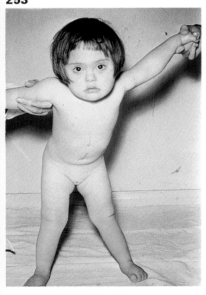

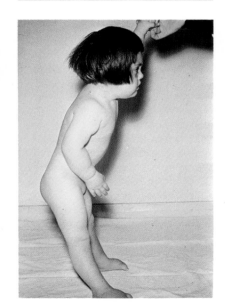

NUTRITIONAL DISORDERS

Nutritional research has established the *adequate* diet for the maintenance of health and normal function in man. This is of particular importance for the growing child. The well-fed child will be free of deficiency diseases and will acquire good resistance to infections, whereas nutritional deprivation, especially during the early stages of life, will produce alarming defects of physical and intellectual development.

Malnutrition in childhood is perpetuated by carelessness, ignorance, poverty and food rituals more prevalent in underdeveloped countries, but still met in the western world.

The indifference to breastfeeding, the physiological infant feeding, is similarly a peculiar phenomenon in our health-conscious age. Inability to breastfeed is rare and contra-indications for mother and child are few. The superiority of breastmilk and the importance of the breastfeeding act is undisputed for the physical and emotional development of the child. Still, over-emphasis on gain in weight soon after birth, misinterpretation of the physiological weight loss and of the transitory hypogalactia at the initiation of lactation, and early complementary feeding are leading causes for unnecessary weaning. The waste of the ideal food for infants is immense, amounting annually to millions of litres.

The decline of breastfeeding has necessitated the search for a suitable substitute. Various attempts to find the ideal formula composition reflect the difficulty experienced with the *humanization* of animal milk.

Nowadays the baby is faced with an abundance of instant milk products, each claiming equality with mother's milk. However, in spite of substantial advances, nutritional breakdowns occur with artificial feeding which lacks the *biological value* of breastmilk. Moreover, the common formula is not individually adapted to the infant's digestive capacity, and is liable to inaccurate preparation.

Unfavourable reports from developing countries where breastfeeding has been rapidly declining have stimulated scientific and popular interest in breastfeeding in the Western world.

New studies have again established breastmilk as the simplest and safest infant food, superior to host defence and the infant's physical and emotional development.

The widespread establishment of breastmilk banks in neonatal units, the arrangements for the collection and storing of expressed breastmilk and antenatal propaganda for breastfeeding point to firmer rooting of this physiological process.

In the older child the preference for sweet foods with a high carbo-hydrate and a relatively low protein content tends to promote rapid gain in weight and obesity with its untoward consequences. Coupled with a low calorie intake irreparable damage may occur.

On the curative side impressive results have been achieved with elimination diets in cases of intestinal malabsorption and in inborn errors of metabolism. The early introduction of these diets prevents the accumulation of toxic split products of nutrients which cannot be further metabolised.

Close supervision is needed to avoid nutritional deficiencies during their prolonged use.

Feeding difficulties developing soon after birth require exclusion of organic causes.

MALNUTRITION

Insufficient calorie intake (254-259)

254 Inanition despite adequate lactation. The breasts are engorged and the flattened nipples make sucking difficult. The 6-week-old baby is wasted, weighing only $2\frac{1}{4}$kg.

255 Dystrophy The 8-week-old infant was artificially fed on a low calorie diet. Note the scaphoid (*hunger*) abdomen, and lack of subcutaneous fat tissue.

256 Marasmus (infantile atrophy) A 2-year-old Asian child with longstanding malnutrition. There is abdominal distension and severe lack of subcutaneous fat tissue, especially in the face, thorax and legs. Note the abundance of hair and the sad depressed attitude.

254

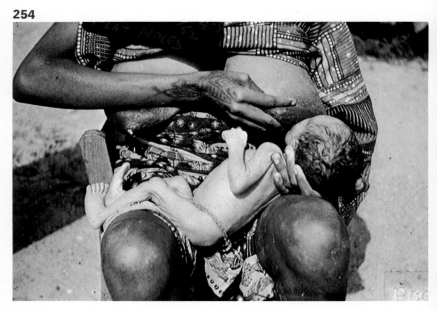

255

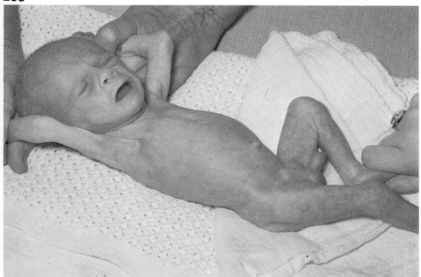

256

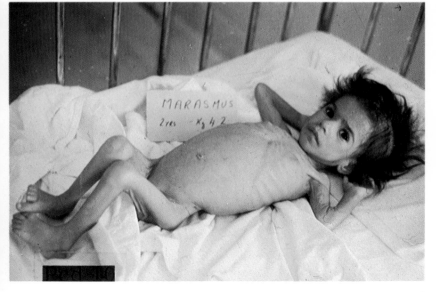

MARASMUS
2 res — Kg 4.2

257 Marasmus The 3-year-old was kept on a low calorie, predominantly carbohydrate diet which led to retention of electrolytes and fluid. Oedema and abdominal distension conceal the poor condition. The child's apathy is obvious.

258 Kwashiorkor A malnutrition due to protein-calorie deficient diet. The predominant features of the syndrome are oedema, a thin peeling skin, reddish discoloration of the hair and lack of emotional reactions. This type of malnutrition occurs mainly in socially and economically under-developed countries.

259 Kwashiorkor and marasmus The $2\frac{1}{2}$-year-old boy on the left has kwashiorkor; the $4\frac{1}{2}$-year-old boy on the right has severe marasmus; the child in the centre is a healthy 2-year-old. The affected children are wasted, oedematous and miserable. The marantic boy is of the same height as the other children although 2 years older. Retardation of growth is common in malnutrition.

257

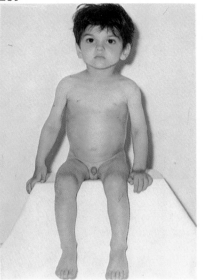

258

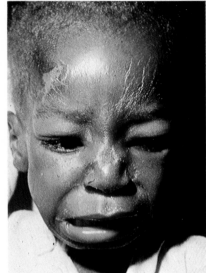

259

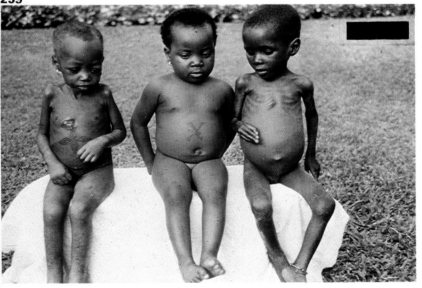

Overfeeding causes less concern as it accelerates growth and development. However, wrong dietary habits in childhood tend to perpetuate into adulthood where the border-line with constitutional obesity and its metabolic and cardiovascular complications is vague.

260 Overhydration (nutritional hydrolability) Girl of 2 months, weight 5500g (*75th centile for 4 months*). Birthweight was 3200g. The feeding formula contained excess of carbohydrates, and lack of protein, leading to increased fluid retention and apparent plumpness easily lost during intercurrent illnesses.

261 Calorie excess Girl of 4 months, weight 9070g (*75th centile for 9 months*). Birthweight was 3850g. Overfeeding was the only cause of the excess deposition of adipose tissue on the face, buttocks and limbs and the cushingoid appearance. The increased cellularity and cell size of the fat tissue which develop in overweight infants seem to reflect unfavourably on obesity in later life (*see* **303-305**).

262 Precocious development Girl aged 10 years. Weight 65kg, height 165cm, corresponding to the 75th centile for 15 years. The distribution of fat tissue on the breasts and abdomen with relatively slim limbs is of adult type. The girl was a compulsive eater (*hyperphagic*).

260

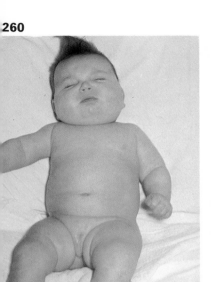

261

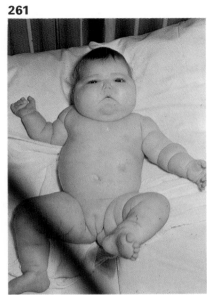

262

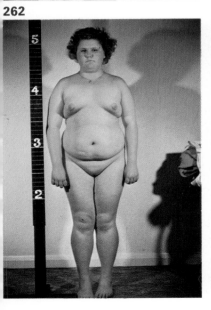

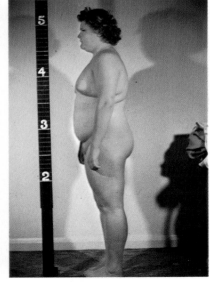

REGURGITATION AND VOMITING

Rumination (merycism) (263-266) A psychosomatic disorder in emotionally disturbed infants. Food is regurgitated and partly re-swallowed after chewing. In severe cases the loss of nutrients can be considerable. Organic causes, e.g. hiatus hernia, must be excluded.

263 Clinical picture At 14 months the girl shows the characteristic physical and emotional behaviour pattern. She is withdrawn and depressed, the gaze is vacant. Note the scaphoid abdomen and infantile flexure posture.

264 & 265 Behaviour during feeding is passive and disinterested (**264**). The abdomen and diaphragm are drawn in, food is regurgitated and re-chewed with obvious lack of discomfort (**265**).

263

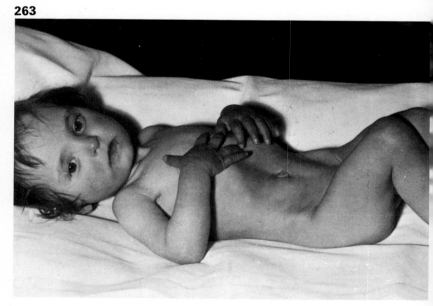

264

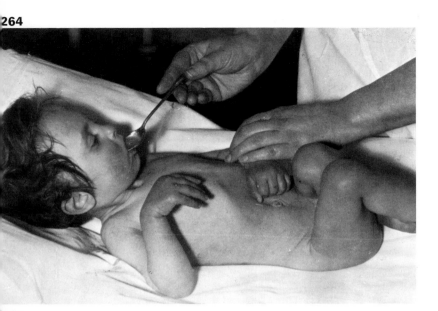

265

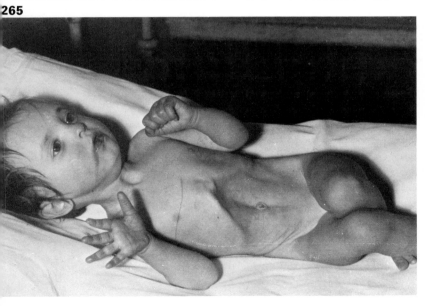

173

266 Withdrawing into solitude with clasped hands the child is sucking her arm, oblivious of the surroundings.

267 Pyloric stenosis A neuro-muscular dysfunction leading to pylorospasm, muscular hypertrophy, gastric dilatation, projectile vomiting and wasting. The abdomen of a 3-month-old infant shows epigastric distension and peristaltic waves. Mild cases recover with conservative treatment, but Weber-Ramstedt operation (*division of the pyloric tumour*) is the treatment of choice.

266

267

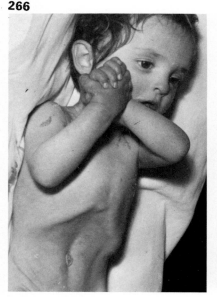
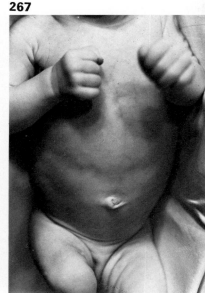

MALABSORPTION

Malabsorption disorders are temporary or permanent disturbances of the digestion and assimilation of essential nutrients.

POSTINFECTIVE

268 Postinfective malabsorption This 5-month-old infant failed to thrive and developed abdominal distension and steatorrhoea. Wasting became severe. The condition gradually resolved with dietetic adjustments using a median-chain trigliceride formula.

268

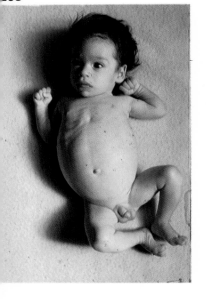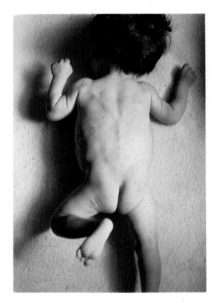

COELIAC

Coeliac disease (269-274) is a specific, genetic enteropathy, often familial. Sensitization by some proteins, mainly by the gliadin component of wheat, and less commonly, by β-lactoglobulin of cow's milk is pathogenic. Changes in the intestinal mucosa particularly affect the absorption of long-chain fatty acids. Irritability, bulky steatorrhoea and wasting ensue.

Apart from clinical signs and duodenal biopsy, a test showing blood xylose values under 20mg/100ml one hour after ingestion of 5gm D-xylose may indicate the presence of the condition.

269 Clinical picture The characteristic appearance is seen in this 4-year-old boy. The face is relatively normal in contrast to the extreme wasting of the body, especially of buttocks and limbs. The grossly distended and overhanging abdomen (*pseudo-ascites*) adds to the grotesque appearance. Height (*86cm*) and weight (*9.5kg*) was below the 3rd centile. Sensitivity to cow's milk could be established.

270 After 6 months considerable improvement is seen. Breastmilk was included in the treatment.

269

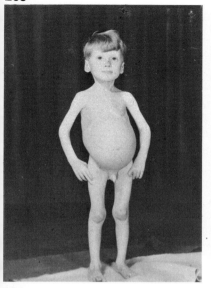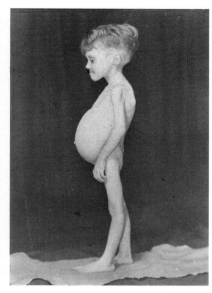

270

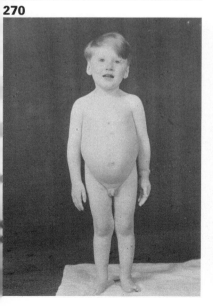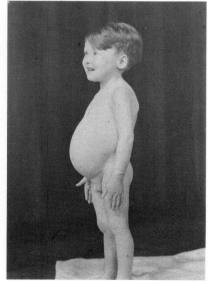

271 Normal development at 23 years. Height 187.6cm, weight 60kg. Short relapses occurred during intercurrent infections.

271

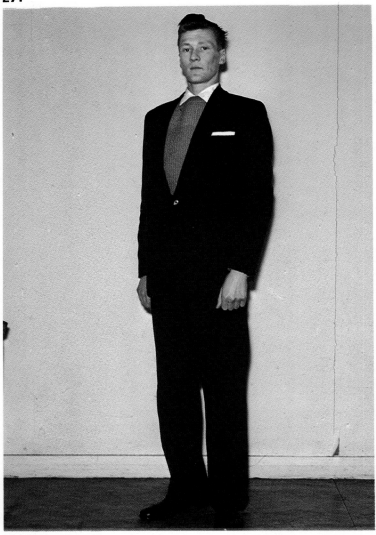

275

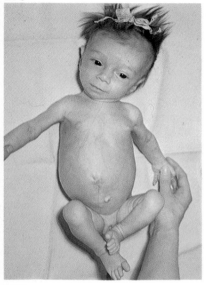

276

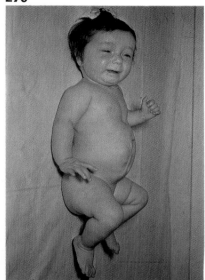

277

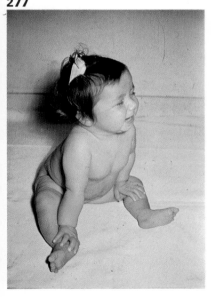

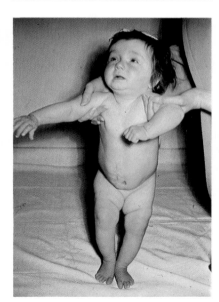

278 Manifestations in the older child are recurrent attacks of chest infection and steatorrhoea. The diagnosis in the 5-year-old boy was confirmed by positive sweat test and trypsin assay from the faeces. Note the pallor and 'wet' appearance of mucous membranes.

279 & 280 Appearance at 9 years General development is retarded. Weight and height remained at the 3rd centile. Discoloration around the eyes, nasal obstruction with open mouth breathing simulate adenoidal features.

281 Clubbing of fingers developed with repeated chest infections. The boy died a few months later.

278

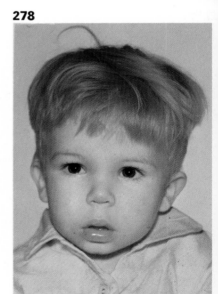

279

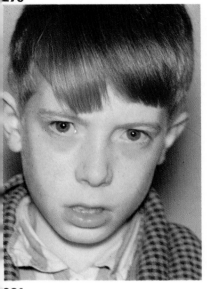

280

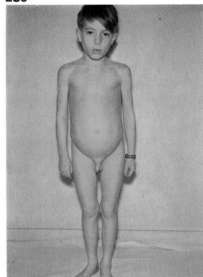

281

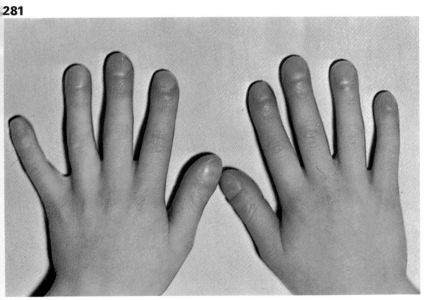

ENZYME DEFECTS

PHENYLKETONURIA

Phenylketonuria (282-285) is an autosomal recessive disorder of protein metabolism. Conversion of phenylalanine into tyrosine is inhibited through deficient activity of phenylalanine hydroxylase. The resulting high blood level of phenylalanine, with its toxic effect on the central nervous system, leads to progressive mental retardation and neurological and general disorders. Phenylpyruvic acid and its metabolites appear in the urine above normal concentration.

The disorder is the leading detectable condition in the communal neonatal screening programme for inborn errors of metabolism enabling successful preventive dietary treatment.

The disorder is the leading detectable condition in the communal neonatal screening programme for inborn errors of metabolism enabling successful preventive dietary treatment by restricting the daily intake of phenylalanine.

282 & 283 Clinical picture The 8-month-old boy referred for refractory eczema, convulsions and lack of intellectual progress, shows the appearance of an attractive, blond, blue-eyed child (*decreased pigmentation*) with mild eczema and hypertonus. He functioned at a 3-months level. Plasma phenylalanine level was 30mg/100ml.

284 & 285 Another case The 2-year-old boy had tremor and convulsion from the age of 6 months (*a 10-year-old sister in a mental home was subsequently diagnosed as affected*), and typical colouring, freckles and patches of eczema. Note the catatonic posture and spasm of the fingers at play. Plasma phenylalanine level was 25mg/100ml. The child improved considerably on a low phenylalanine diet.

Normal intellectual development can be expected if dietary treatment is started during the first two months of life. Delayed start can result in irreversible brain damage.

After terminating the dietary restrictions repeated monitoring of IQ should be carried out. With few exceptions affected children will show a decline in performance.

There is a strong case for low-phenylalanine diet during the pregnancy of phenylketonuric mothers. Otherwise perinatal complications and malformations may occur.

(*Conditions of enzyme defects with severe skeletal dysplasias are presented on pages 326-331.*)

282

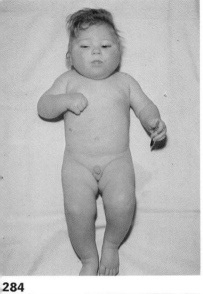

283

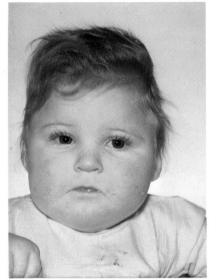

284

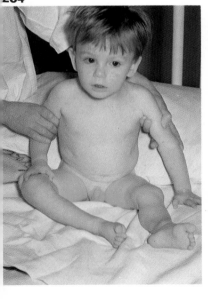

285

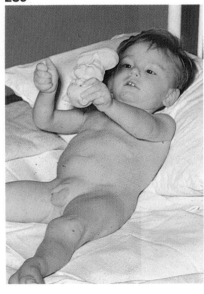

THE OBESE CHILD

This is a serious, complex disorder prone to relapses and refractory to treatment. Genetic factors, social conditions, anxiety and tension are contributory. Studies of the cellular composition of adipose tissue has thrown a new light on the understanding of this condition.

286 & 287 Postural defects in obesity The 3-year-old boy shows valgus deformity of the legs and lordosis, which may persist throughout life.

286

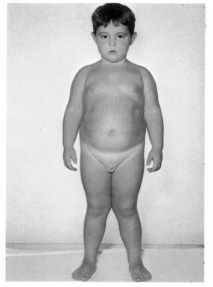
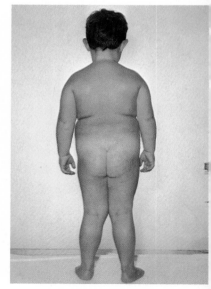

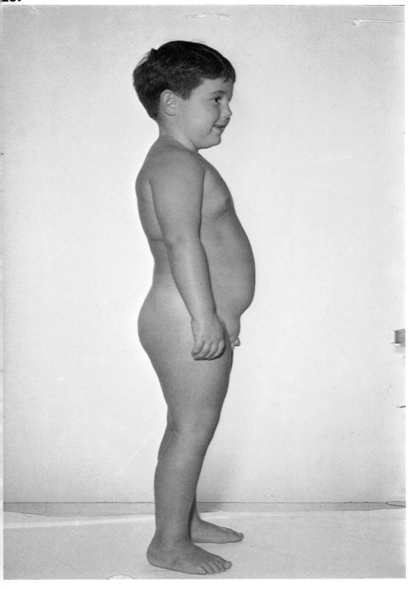

288 Similarity of appearance in a 7-year-old boy and 9-year-old girl. The likeness of obese children, irrespective of relation or sex, is demonstrated. Both children show a high-coloured face and buttocks, signs of minor hypercorticism. The hormonal assay is usually normal.

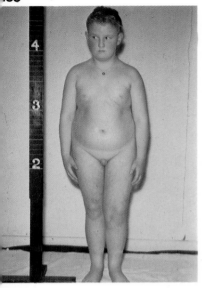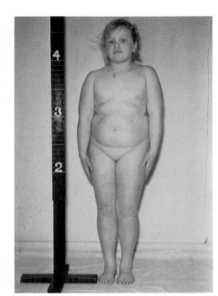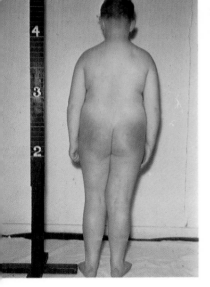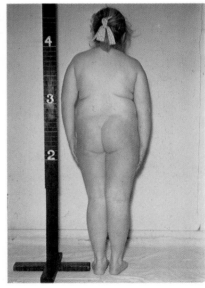

289-291 Rapid development of secondary sex characteristics, a high-coloured face and striae, are seen in this 11-year-old obese girl. This may lead to embarrassment and behaviour difficulties.

289

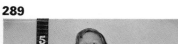

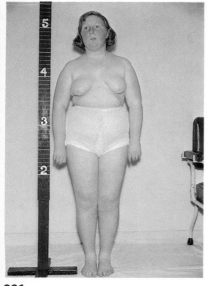

290

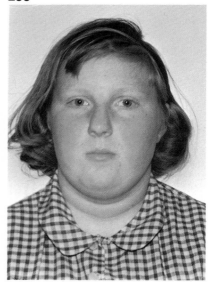

291

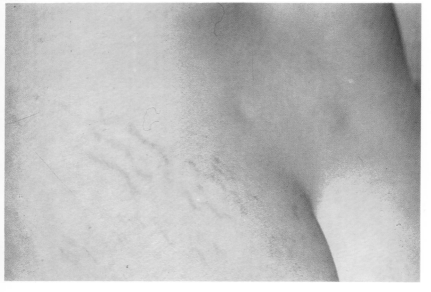

193

292 & 293 Pseudo-hypogenitalism in a 10-year-old boy. In contrast to the female child, the obese male shows apparent hypogenitalism due to excessive pubic fat deposition, and a feminine aspect of adiposity. Note the apron-like overhanging abdomen (*hottentot abdomen*).

292

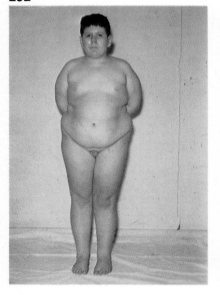 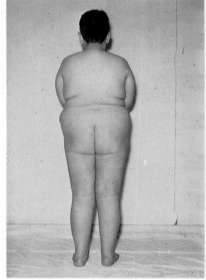

194

293

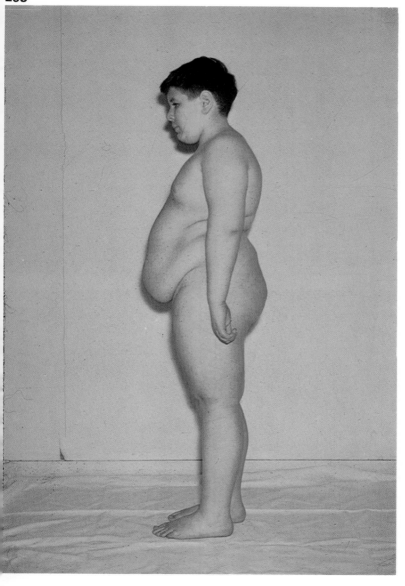

294 & 295 Hereditary predisposition These obese siblings show a similar distribution of subcutaneous fat tissue and signs of mild hypercorticism. The 17-hydroxy-corticosteroid level was slightly elevated.

296 Obese girl and normal child of the same age Weight difference was 15.25kg. Note the difference in height.

294

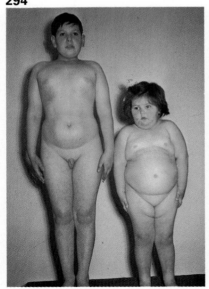

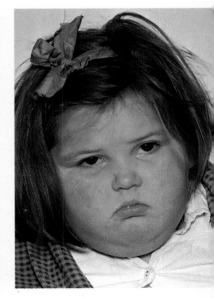

295

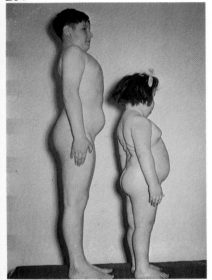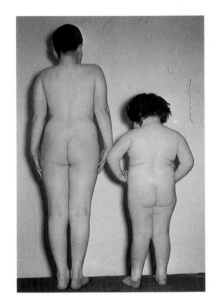

296

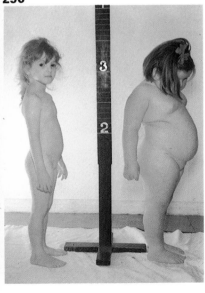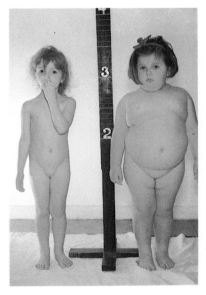

197

297 Maladjustment This grossly obese girl of 11 years shows the influence of emotional factors. Coming from an insecure family background she was depressed and an obsessional eater.

298 & 299 Rehabilitation Later at the age of 20 years, married to a 50-year-old father figure, and after birth of a child, her appearance had changed to normal.

297

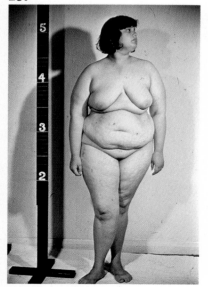
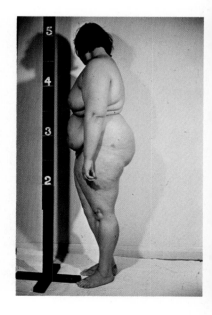

298

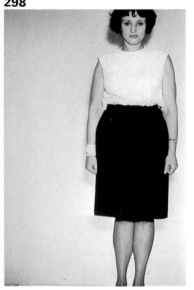
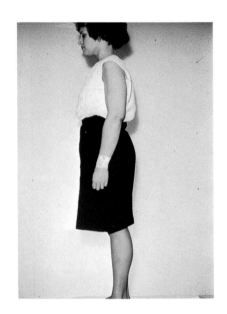

299

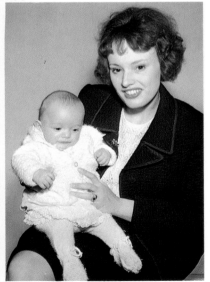

300-302 Mid-childhood obesity (300) tends to improve at puberty in both sexes **(301 & 302)**.

300

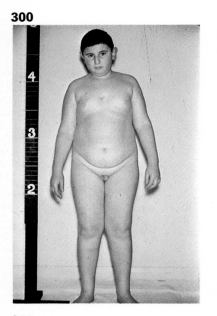 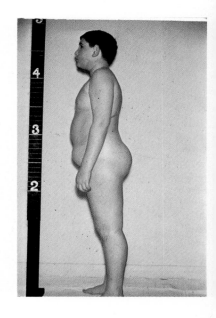

301

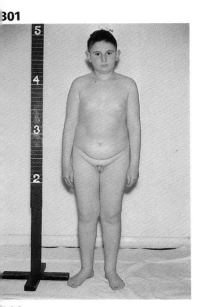
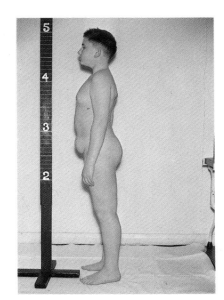

302

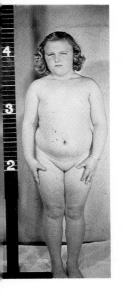
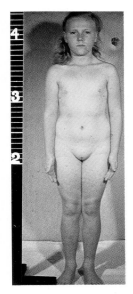

303-305 Early childhood obesity is likely to persist. Note the condition at the age of 14 months (**303**) and the further deterioration in stages at the age of 5 years (**304**), 8 years and 14 years (**305**) to reach Pickwickian proportions.

303

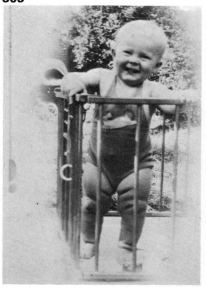

304

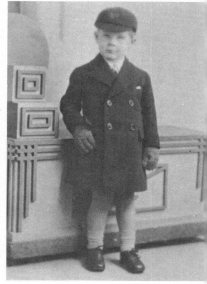

305

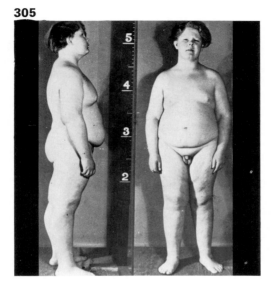

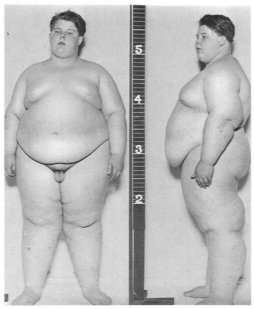

THE LEAN CHILD

There are constitutionally lean, healthy children, who remain so in adulthood. Malnutrition, psychological disorders and the diencephalic syndrome have to be excluded.

306 & 307 Pseudo-cachexia The weight of the 8-year-old boy was on the 3rd centile for chronological height. The lateral view underlines the slim features of the body. The 9-year-old girl was more severely affected (**307**). She developed emotional problems because of her appearance. Increased calorie intake was not effective.

308 Progressive lipodystrophy A condition with insidious loss of adipose tissue from the upper part of the body. The 10-year-old girl shows the classical appearance : a lined face, thin arms and chest. In contrast the lower normal body appears hypertrophic. These features persist throughout life and are only amenable to plastic surgery.

306

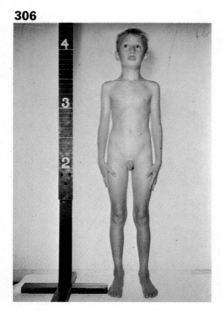
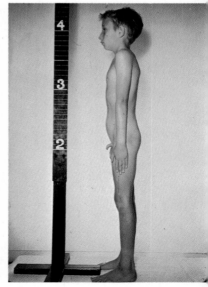

307

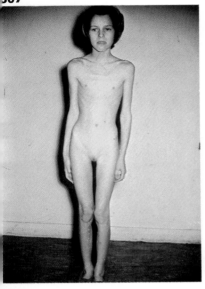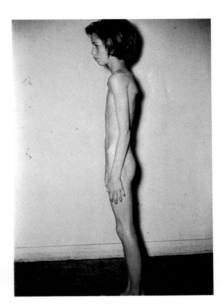

308

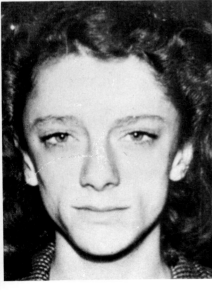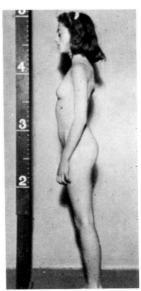

THE SMALL CHILD (DWARFISM)

Stunted growth implies the retardation of linear growth below the accepted norm. There is a broad spectrum of causes and phenotypes, some easily discernible by the presence of particular malformations or by the child's peculiar appearance. In less obvious cases the evaluation of the family pattern, diseases, environmental conditions and finally the hormonal assay will decide the prognosis and therapeutic approach.

Idiopathic non-hormonal dwarfism is shown in three cases:

309 Nanism (ateleiosis), familial short stature The 2-year-old girl is shown with a normal sized child of the same age. The parents and four siblings were short. Note the well developed, proportionate body. The bone age and intellectual development were normal. The child's height observed over a period of 3 years remained below the 3rd centile.

309

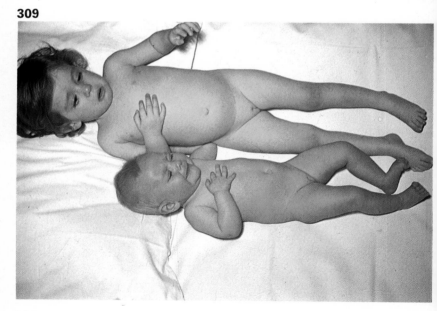

310-312 Silver-Russel dwarfism without asymmetry The appearance at 14 months (310). The girl, seen with her normal sized 9-year-old brother and 10-year-old sister, is of midget size. The birth-weight (*2000g*) was low for her normal gestational age. At 14 months her height (*61cm*) had reached only the 3rd centile for an age of 6 months.

310

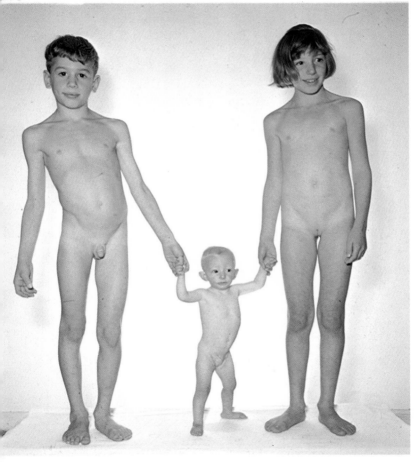

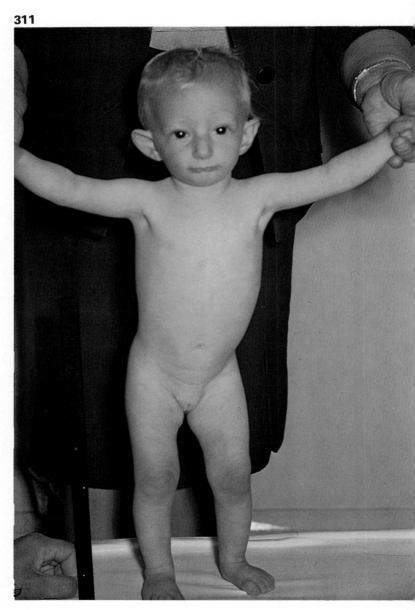

311 & 312 Characteristic features Note the bossing forehead, the triangular face small in proportion to the skull, the large eyes, protruding large ears and the hypoplastic receding chin.

The body is symmetrical and proportionate, and the neuromuscular development and intelligence were adequate for age. The plasma growth hormone level was normal. Apart from an accessory 6th finger (removed) and a low left kidney there was no clinical or test evidence of any other defect.

312

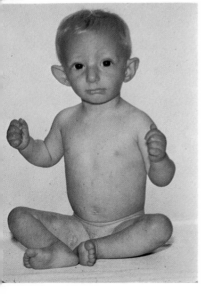
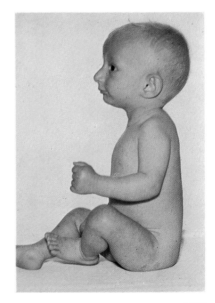

313 Primordial idiopathic dwarfism observed over a period of 6 years. Birthweight at 37 weeks' gestation was 1500g, length 42cm, increasing to 51cm at 6 months (*top, left*) and to 57cm at 1 year (*top, right*), the 25th centile for 3 months. The appearance hardly changed during that time.

At 3 years (*bottom, left*) compared with a normal control, the infantilism is marked. Height was 65.9cm, the 3rd centile for 15 months.

At 6 years (*bottom, right*) the dwarfism was progressive. Height was 80.6cm, the 3rd centile for 3 years (*normal height would have been 114.6cm*). No evidence of hypopituitarism was detected and the plasma growth hormone level was normal.

(*For other forms of dwarfism see* **Skeletal Dysplasias,** *page 322.*)

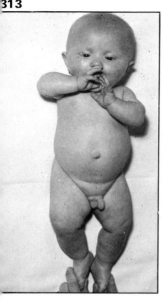
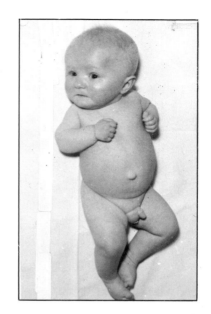
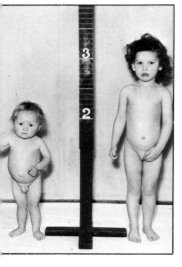
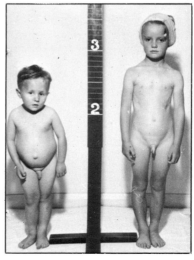

THE ALLERGIC CHILD

Allergic manifestations are the result of antigen-antibody interaction in a sensitized individual. Sensitization could have occurred either transplacentally or by inhalation, ingestion or contact with, an antigen. The tendency to react is inherited and often a familial pattern is repeated in the child. Some common manifestations are shown.

SKIN ALLERGY

314 & 315 Urticaria The face, arms and legs are covered with bright red wheals which are waxing and waning. There is conjunctivitis and oedema of the face and lips. The child protects his inflamed eyes against the light. Eggs were the antigenic agent.

316 Papular urticaria Common especially in the spring. A follicular eruption developing into hard itchy vesicles. Differentiate from varicella. (*see* **358 & 359**).

314

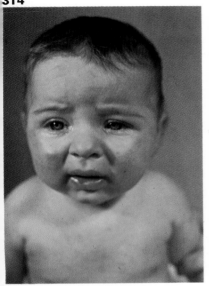

315

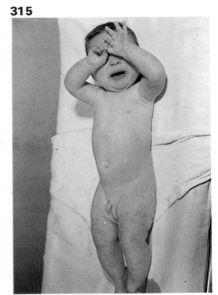

316

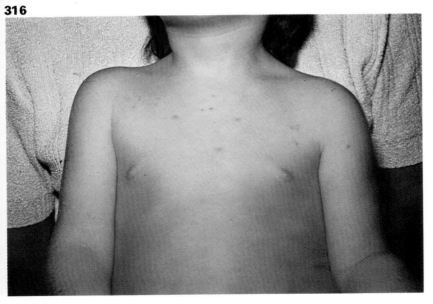

Atopic dermatitis (317-319) There are two types of manifestation during childhood, characterised by intense itching. A multiplicity of causative agents, including imbalanced function of the autonomic system, has been postulated.

317 Infantile eczema appears early in infancy with variable severity and persistence. There is erythema and oozing with the formation of crusts which can affect the whole body. It is intensified by rubbing. The localization on the face and arms, the parts exposed to light, indicates the cause of sensitization in this case.

318 & 319 Neurodermatitis A widespread disorder of older children. The face shows crusty blepharitis, eczema on the cheeks, cracked dry lips with cheilitis and perlèche.

Dry, scaly or inflamed, and later oozing patches appear (**319**). Lichenification in the elbow and knee flexures (*flexural pruritus*) occurs simultaneously and is usually longlasting. The 5-year-old girl is covered with eruptions and excoriations, the result of the itch-scratch cycle.

A reaction to insect bites or scabies, and to metabolic disorders (*see* **282-285**) has to be excluded.

317

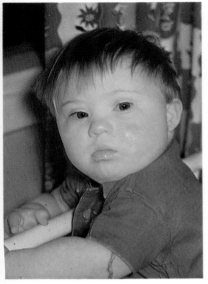

318

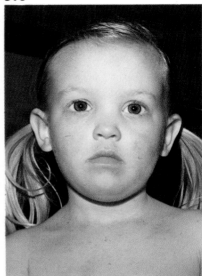

319

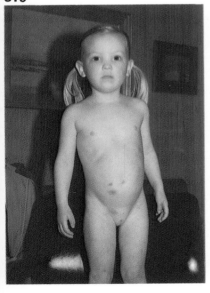

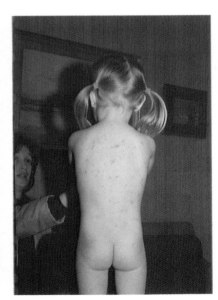

Complications are produced by bacterial or viral superinfection.

320 Impetiginized facial eczema A pyogenic staphylococcal or streptococcal infection. Note the honey-coloured crusts and the poor state of general health. The infection is nephrotoxic, particularly in younger children.

321 Eczema herpeticum A superinfection with herpes or coxsackie virus.

322-324 Eczema vaccinatum (Kaposi's varicelliform eruption) Atopic dermatitis infected with vaccinia virus by contact with a recently vaccinated sister. The face and legs are covered with haemorrhagic crusts. In the cubital flexures and on the left thigh are fresh pustular eruptions (**324**). A dangerous complication requiring hospitalisation (*see* **358 & 359**).

320

321

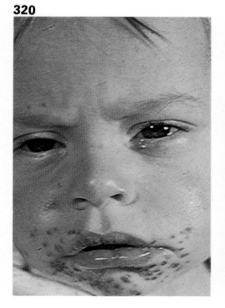
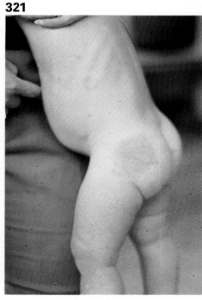

322

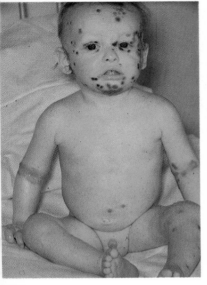

323

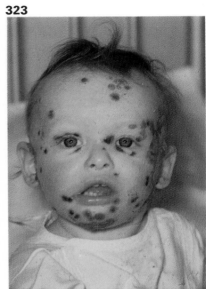

324

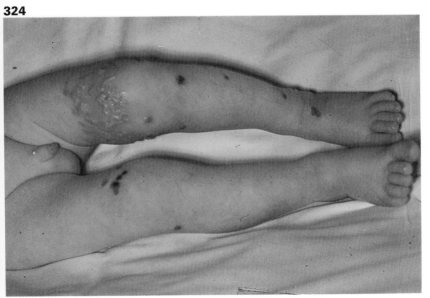

RESPIRATORY ALLERGY

Allergic perennial rhinitis (325-328) often occurs with attacks of asthma or spasmodic bronchitis. A common manifestation in early childhood.

325 & 326 Clinical picture The 5-year-old girl shows infraorbital oedema and a gaping mouth, a sign of nasal obstruction by hypertrophic lymphoid tissue. Note the large fleshy tonsils and the *geographical tongue* (**326**). The changing pattern of desquamation and epithelial thickening persists throughout life (*see* **615**).

327 & 328 Reactions to itching The child develops typical mannerisms like rubbing the nose laterally with one finger or pushing it upwards with the flat palm, in order to relieve the itching.

325

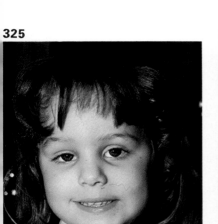

326

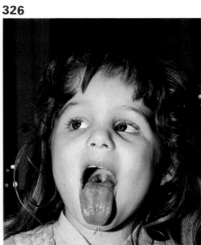

327

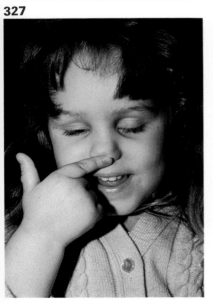

328

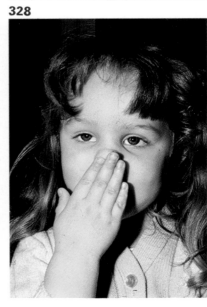

329 Hay fever, atopic rhinitis A non-infective condition of seasonal occurrence frequently associated in childhood with atopic dermatitis. Note the pallor, the discoloration of the lower palpebral area, the mucoid nasal discharge and oedema of the lips.

329

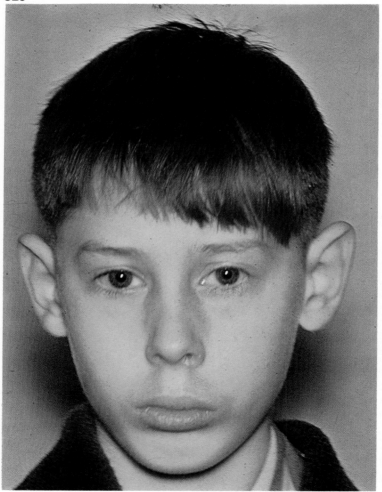

DISEASES

COLLAGEN (AUTO-IMMUNE) DISEASES

A variety of acute and chronic diseases are grouped together because of similar connective tissue lesions, possibly related to auto-immunisation.

Rheumatic fever (330-333) usually appears in the trait of infections with Lancefield group A β-haemolytic streptococci.

330 Erythema nodosum rheumaticum heralds the disease. Reddish-blue painful nodules of various size appear on the anterior aspect of the tibiae.

330

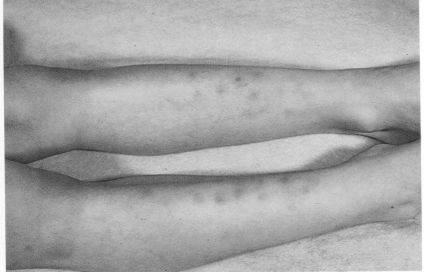

331 Polyarthritis follows, involving the larger joints. This 8-year-old boy displays the symmetrical swellings of shoulder, wrist and ankle joints (*in contrast to rheumatoid arthritis which is asymmetrical and affects the small joints*).

332 & 333 Close-up of the swollen wrists and ankles The widespread erythematous macular rash and jaundice is a toxic-allergic reaction to salicylates.

331

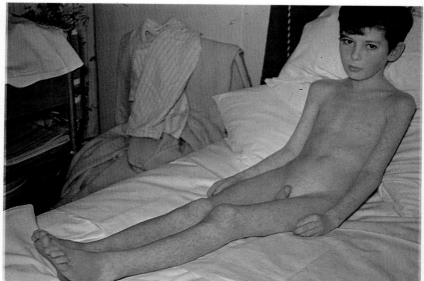

332

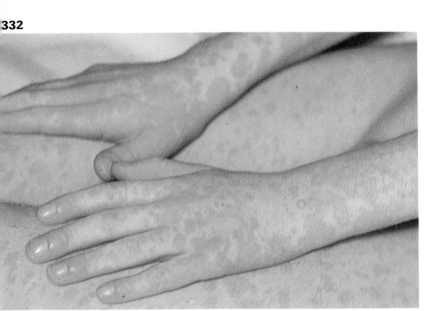

333

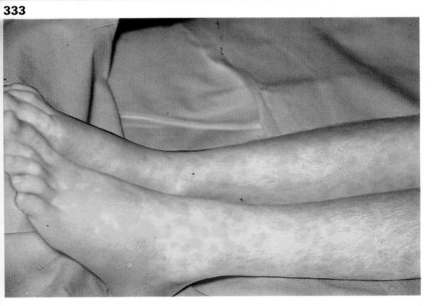

334 Anaphylactoid purpura (Schönlein-Henoch) A hypersensitivity reaction to streptococcal infections and other causes with capillary damage involving the skin, joints and kidneys. It is liable to recur. The prognosis depends on the degree and persistence of renal involvement. This 3-year-old boy fell acutely ill with joint and abdominal pain, and haematuria. Note the distribution of the macular purpuric rash on the limbs and buttocks. The face and trunk remain free.

335 Papular purpura A variant of the manifestation.

336 Idiopathic thrombocytopenic purpura The disease, probably of auto-immune origin, is triggered off by infections or sensitizing agents (*drugs*), leading to increased platelet destruction and haemorrhage. The 5-year-old girl, seen here in an attack, had intermittent epistaxis, petechiae and bruising from the age of 2 years. Her face and limbs are covered with large bruises. Recovery followed splenectomy.

334

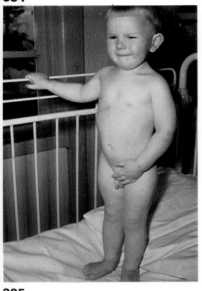
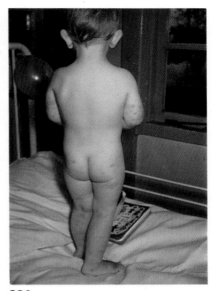

335

336

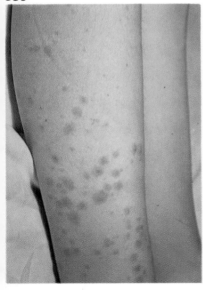
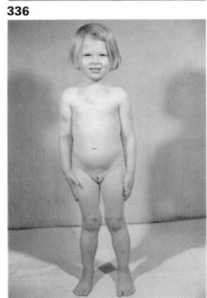

337-339 Acute thrombocytopenic purpura due to aspirin-induced platelet dysfunction (*aggregation defect*). The 18-month-old boy received a total of 150mg acetylsalicylic acid. The striking picture of the purpuric rash covering the face, limbs and buttocks was self-limiting and faded within one week.

340 Erythema multiforme circinata A rash of widespread distribution consisting of raised, circumscribed erythematous areas with central blanching, associated with infections or connective tissue diseases. It is self-limiting, but tends to recur.

337

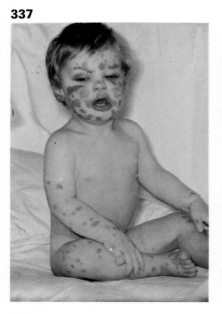

338

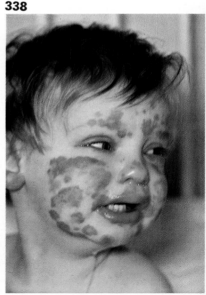

339

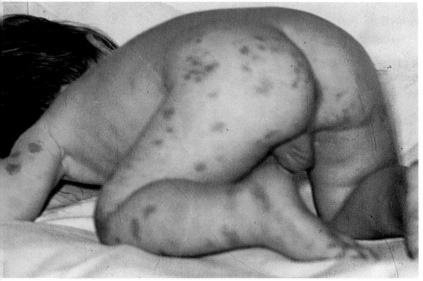

340

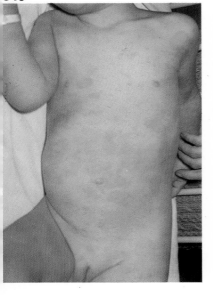
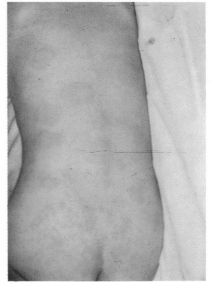

THE IDIOPATHIC NEPHROTIC SYNDROME
(*LIPOID NEPHROSIS*)

A sensitivity reaction to an ill-defined allergen affecting kidney function and morphology connected with generalised oedema, proteinuria, disturbance of the serum protein composition and elevation of the cholesterol level.

The prognosis depends upon the degree of glomerular involvement ascertained by percutane kidney biopsy.

341 Onset of the disease The 7-year-old girl developed oedema and oliguria over several weeks.

342-345 Treatment with daily steroid regime reduced the oedema, but produced severe side effects of cushingoid appearance and alopecia. The renal function and plasma values became normal. A slight *residual proteinuria* persisted for some time.

341

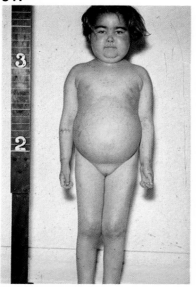
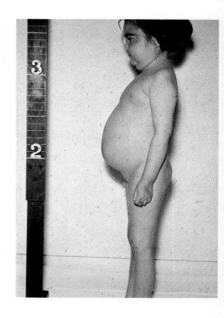

342

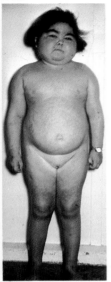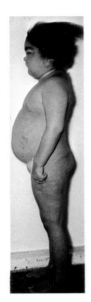

343

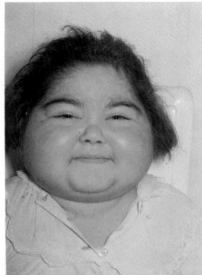

344

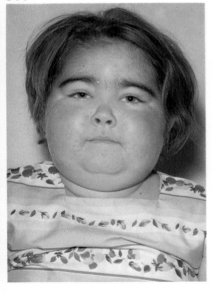

345

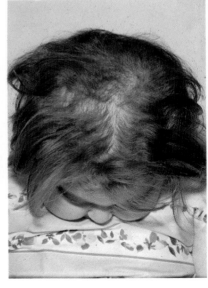

346 Remission One year after cessation of treatment the steroid side-effects are regressing.

347 & 348 Alternate day steroid regime Only minimal cushingoid changes developed in this 5-year-old boy. The growth was not retarded.

346

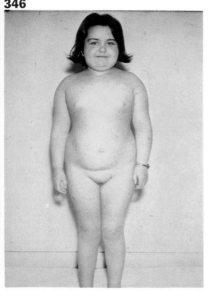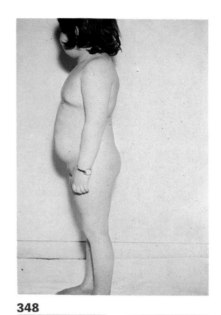

347

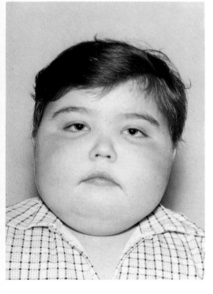

348

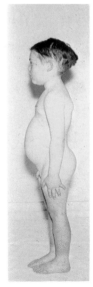

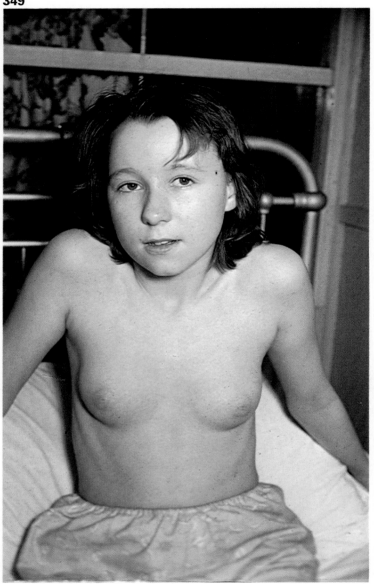

349 Scarlet fever is caused by infection with haemolytic streptococci. The bright red punctate rash starts in the face and spreads downwards. The perioral area remains free (*circumoral pallor*).

350 & 351 The characteristic changes in the tongue produced by desquamation of the initially furred tongue (*white strawberry tongue* **350**) and swelling of the papillae (*red strawberry tongue* **351**).

350

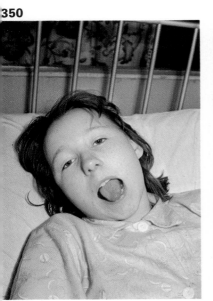

351

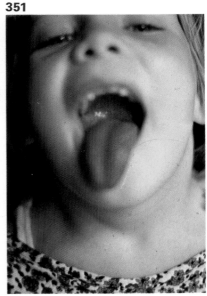

352 & 353 Measles (morbilli) The 6-year-old girl was in contact with measles 10 days earlier. Prodromal signs are furred tongue, high-coloured cheeks, Koplick's spots and enanthema on the oral mucosa.

354 The fully-developed exanthema Note the absence of the rash on parts not exposed to sunlight (*the girl had just returned from a holiday in the sun*).

352

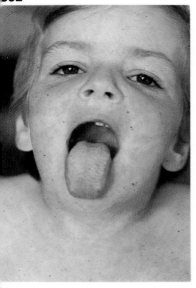

353

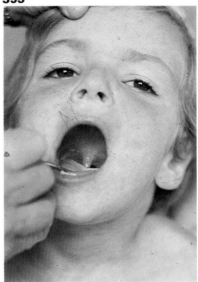

354

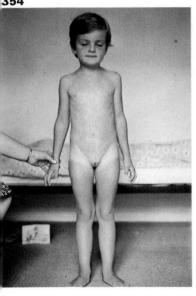

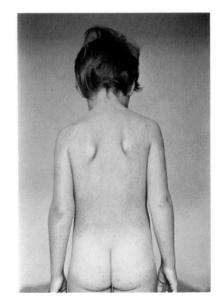

355 Rubella (German measles) Incipient exanthema. A pale pink macular rash on the face and chest. Note the absence of catarrhal signs.

356 The enanthema is confined to the hard and soft palate in contrast to measles where the whole oral mucosa is involved.

357 The discrete pink macular rash is not characteristic. Enlargement of the nuchal lymph glands is diagnostic. In females confirmation by serological test for rubella haemagglutination inhibition (HI) antibodies is advisable in view of future pregnancies (*see* **229-232**).

358 & 359 Varicella (chickenpox) A papular rash turning into clear vesicles. The stages of fresh eruptions and vesicles with scab formations dispersed over the scalp and body are diagnostic (*see* **322-324**).

355

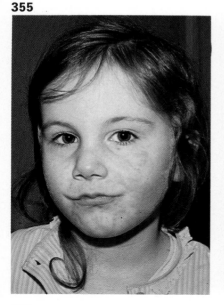

356

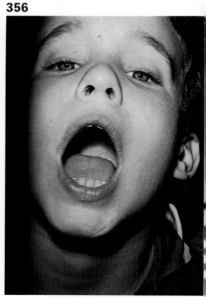

236

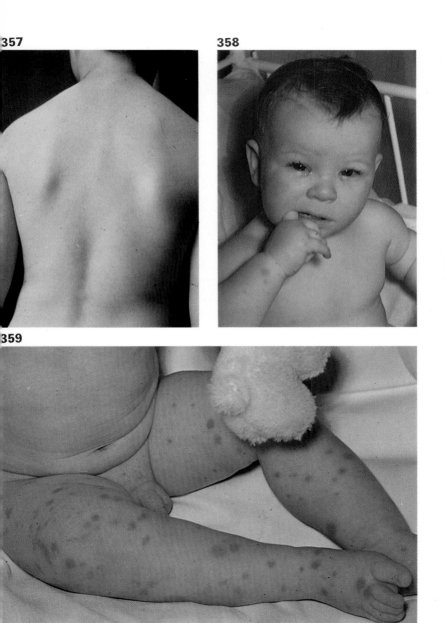

357

358

359

360 Epidemic parotitis (mumps) Unilateral or bilateral swelling develops in the preauricular and submandibular region.

361 The earlobe is displaced upwards and outwards.

362 Viral meningoencephalitis One of the complications of parotitis, usually of benign character. The child is seen in a convulsion.

360

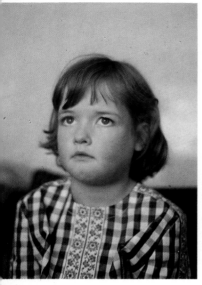

361

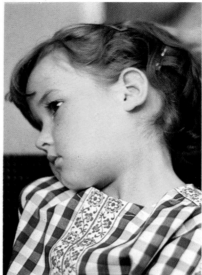

362

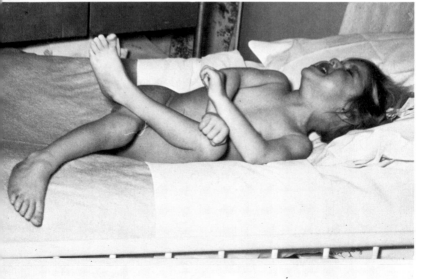

363 & 364 Infectious mononucleosis (glandular fever, Pfeiffer's disease) A polymorph exanthema and jaundice, generalised lymphadenopathy and splenomegaly are the leading signs.

The heterophyl antibody test (*Paul-Bunnel*) was positive (*1:64*). The blood picture would show many mononuclear lymphocytes.

Recently, the disease has been connected with the Epstein-Barr virus.

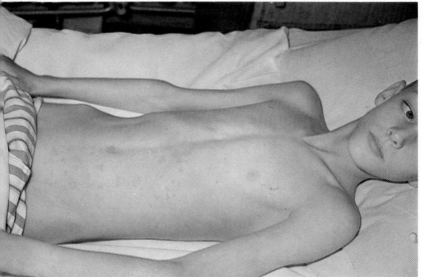

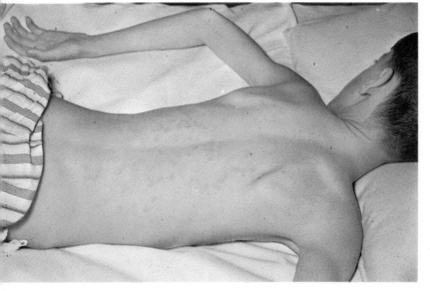

TUBERCULOSIS

The clinical manifestations and the course of this specific infection with the human or bovine type of the acid-fast *mycobacterium tuberculosum* (*Koch*) is influenced by the age, race and social-economic conditions of the patient.

The developing specific allergy and tissue hypersensitivity (*Pirquet*) is detectable by the tuberculin test. This and the isolation of the tubercle bacillus is the principal diagnostic procedure.

The availability of antimicrobial drugs and preventive immunisation has considerably improved the prognosis of this disease.

Diagnostic procedure (365-367)   Performance and evaluation of the Tuberculin tests.

365 Mantoux test This is the most reliable test, performed by intra-cutaneous injection with 0.1cc of a 1:10,000 dilution of Old Tuberculin P.P.D. Read after 24 hours there is erythema without oedema. At this stage the reaction is inconclusive.

366 Read after 48 hours there is a central induration with an erythe-matous halo exceeding 10mm in diameter. The test is positive.

367 Cutaneous Pirquet test Performed with a drop of Old Tuber-culin on the forearm and superficial puncture. The first test seen on the patient's left forearm was negative. Re-testing on the right forearm was inconclusive. The third test performed one week later was positive. Note the flare-up of the older test areas.

For group testing the *Heaf Test* and *Tine Test* are used.

368 Erythema nodosum tuberculosum A tuberculo-toxic sensi-tivity reaction appears simultaneously with the primary infection.

365

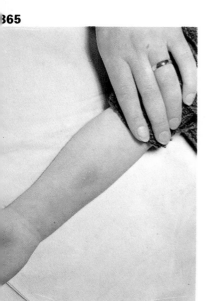

366

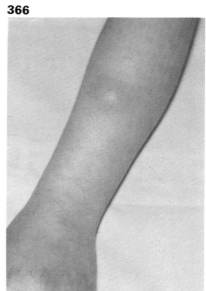

367

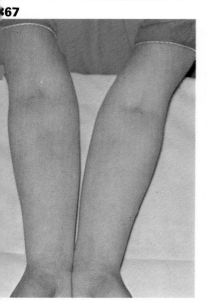

368

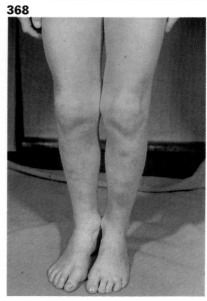

243

369 Respiratory infection The primary complex (*Ranke*) consists of the primary pulmonary lesion (*Ghon focus*), usually situated subpleurally in the right lobe, and the involvement of the hilar glands, which are faintly outlined.

370 A few weeks later during treatment the primary focus has disappeared and the hilar glands are now clearly visible.

371 One year later the glands have regressed leaving an increased hilar shadow. The fine line of interlobar pleurisy on the right indicates the localisation of the primary focus.

369

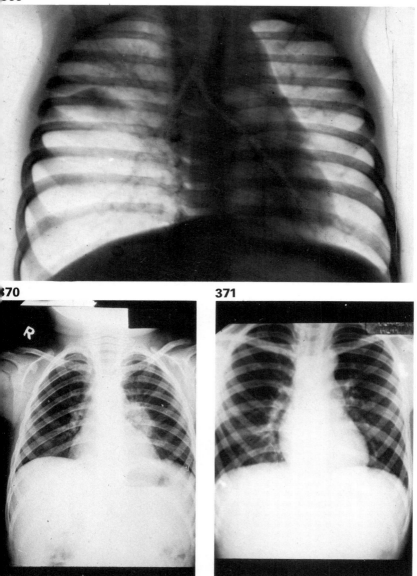

370

371

372 Secondary tuberculosis develops with haematogenic or bronchogenic spread. X-ray film of a case of bilateral tuberculous bronchopneumonia. The mediastinal shift is due to the turning of the neck.

373 Caseous bronchopneumonia and collapse of the right lower lobe. Note the patchy dissemination and the involvement of the hilar glands.

374 Miliary tuberculosis Snow flake appearance of the lung fields. Note the marked mediastinal shift to the right and emphysema due to obstruction and valve action by the hypertrophic tracheobronchial glands.

372

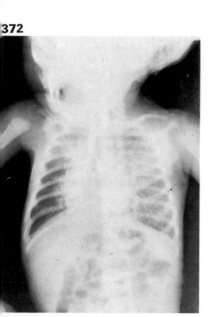

373

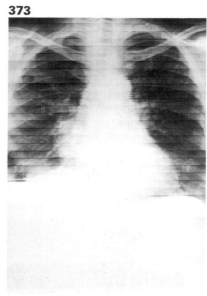

374

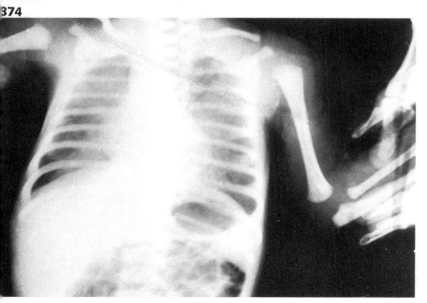

375 & 376 Choroidal tubercles and choked disk A drawing of the ocular fundus of this case. Six months after initiation of treatment (**376**) the lesions have markedly coalesced.

377 Skin infection A 3-month-old baby lived with the grandmother who had a positive sputum.
 A small area of papulo-necrotic tuberculides on the cheek is the primary lesion resulting from the contact.

378 Scrofuloderma and infected caseous inguinal glands The primary focus was found on the cervix.

379 Close-up a few weeks later shows regression on the right side. The area on the left side is still discharging.

375

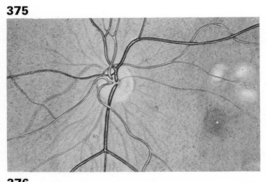

376

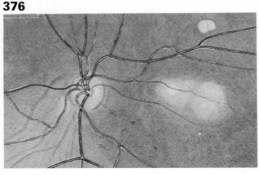

377

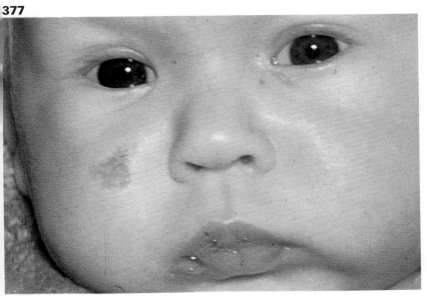

378

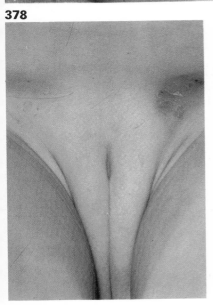

379

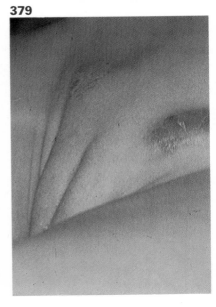

380 Congenital infection Identical twins, 13 years old. The infection was suspected at the age of 6 weeks and was subsequently confirmed in the mother and infants.

The taller twin developed tuberculous meningitis and became a mild spastic. Note the difference in sexual development.

381 Preventive measures Immunisation with the *Bacillus Calmette-Guérin* has spectacularly reduced the incidence and mortality rate of tuberculosis, especially in countries where it is obligatory. The twins shown, whose mother had active tuberculosis, were inoculated at the age of 6 weeks and were isolated until the Mantoux reaction became positive. Then they were returned into mother's care.

Lately a prophylactic course with isoniazid is favoured as this avoids separation.

382 At the age of 1 year the babies showed excellent development and had remained free from tuberculous infection.

380

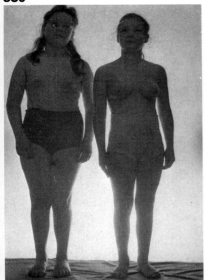

381

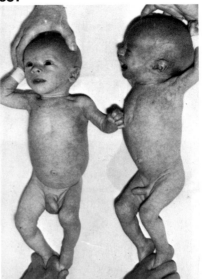

382

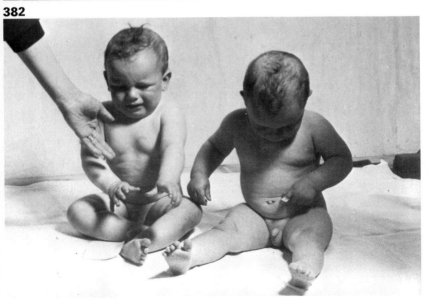

383 Hypochromic iron deficiency anaemia This boy of 7 years developed pallor and lassitude. The blood picture revealed microcytosis, low haematocrit, haemoglobin and serum iron values.

384 & 385 Koilonychia (spoon nails) is occasionally seen in this condition. The nails are concave and split on the edges.

383

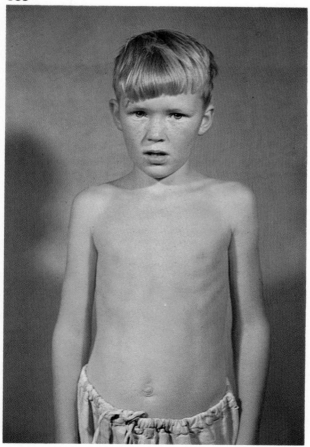

384

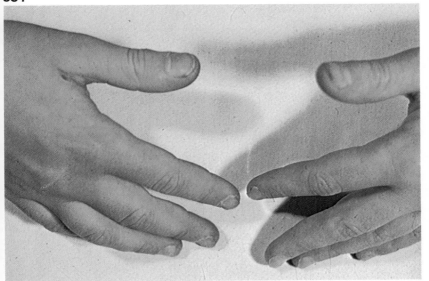

385

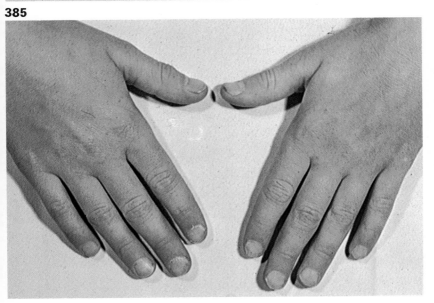

253

386 Thalassaemia major (Cooley's anaemia) A hypochromic anaemia characterised by haemolysis and failure of haemoglobin synthesis of the beta chain. This 2-year-old Negro girl shows the peculiar muddy-icteric colour, bossing forehead and depressed nasal bridge. The prognathia and protruding lips are due to skeletal hypertrophy. Haemosiderosis develops in the course of the frequent transfusions.

387 & 388 Close-ups show very pale palmae and plantae.

386

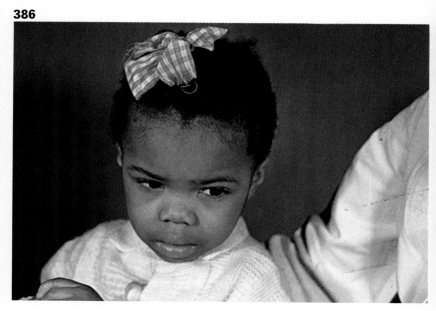

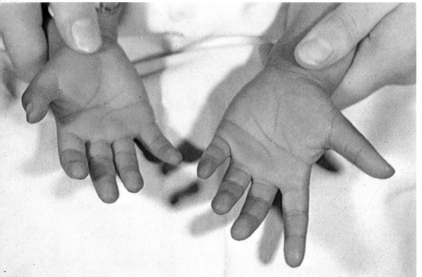

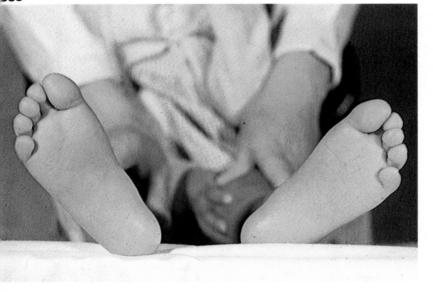

389 Erythrogenesis imperfecta (Diamond-Blackfan syndrome) A congenital progressive hypoplastic anaemia due to defective erythropoiesis. Typical appearance at the age of 2 years showing delicate features, fair hair, pallor and jaundice. The girl had numerous blood transfusions prior to steroid treatment.

390 & 391 At the age of 7 and 8 years the anaemia was controlled with steroid treatment producing increasing side effects. The growth was particularly impaired.

392 At the age of 14 years Comparison with her 6-year-old sister demonstrates the degree of stunted growth. Onset of puberty is delayed. The cushingoid changes have partly receded.

389

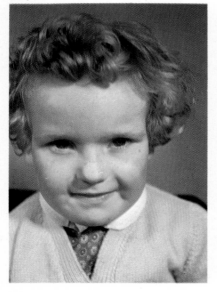

390

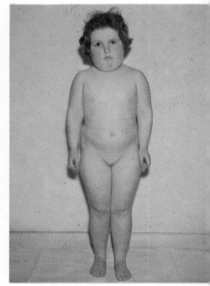

391

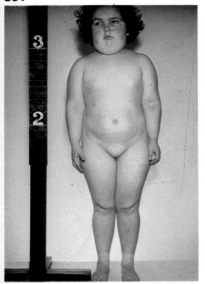
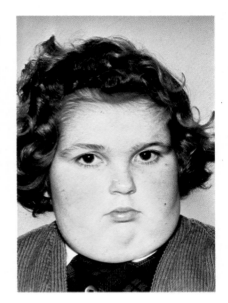

392

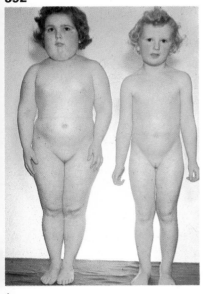

257

ENDOCRINE DISORDERS

THE THYROID GLAND

393 Transitory hypothyroidism Dizygous isosexual twins. The twin on the right developed hypothyroid features, a large protruding tongue and facial oedema. The other twin was normal. The mother was euthyroid and had no antithyroid antibodies.

394 At 10 years he had developed normally without therapy. Immature enzymatic function had led to a temporary block of thyroxin synthesis.

Early recognition and treatment of congenital hypothyroidism (incidence 1:5000) is essential to prevent mental retardation. The disorder should be included in neonatal screening programmes.

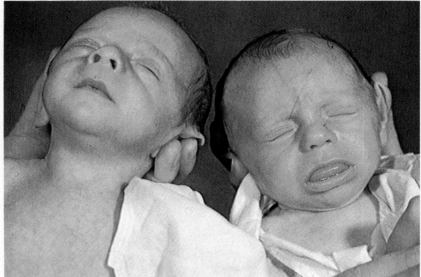

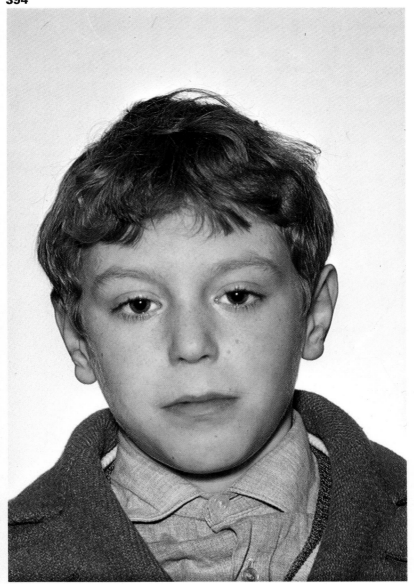

The following two cases show the value of early treatment.

395 Congenital myxoedema The 5-week-old child (*left*) shows generalised myxoedema, dry skin and umbilical hernia. Other signs were a hoarse, low-pitched cry, low body temperature and constipation. With replacement therapy the same child at 2 years shows normal development (*right*).

396 & 397 Another case observed over 11 years The 6-week-old baby is severely affected. Note the marked myxoedema, protruding tongue, distended abdomen and jaundice. The family history was negative.

395

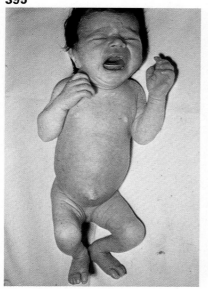
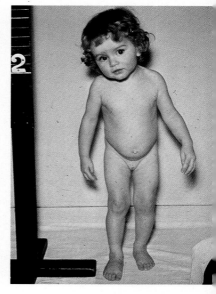

396

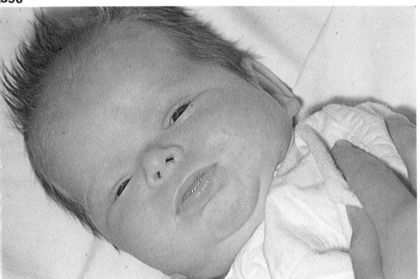

397

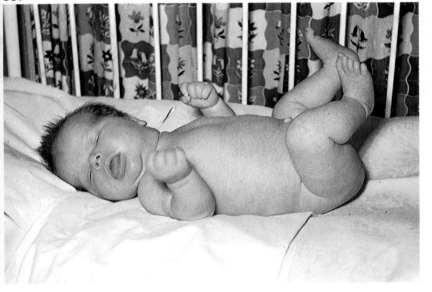

398 & 399 After 3 months of treatment there was considerable improvement in appearance and alertness (*the tongue is coated with monilia*).

400 & 401 At 11 years he had reached normal height and weight. IQ 110.

398

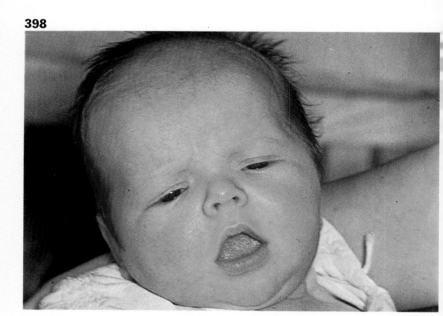

399

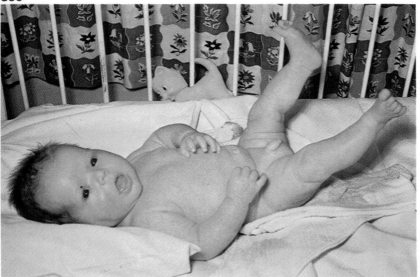

400

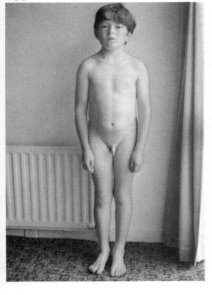

401

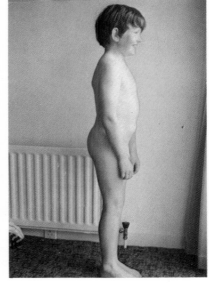

402 Hypothyroidism with residual function This 20-month-old boy had progressed well for 14 months. Then growth stopped and he became slow. X-ray showed retarded bone age. Seen with a normal child the dwarfing is obvious. Note the relatively alert expression and moderate myxoedema. The residual thyroid function had delayed the diagnosis.

403 At 16 years Normal physical and intellectual development was achieved with replacement therapy.

404 Cretin aged 5 years with large goitre Mentally deficient. Several members of the family were similarly affected. They lived in an area where cretinism was endemic.

405 Hyperthyroidism in a 13-day-old infant The mother suffered from Grave's disease and long-acting thyroid stimulator (LATS) activity was transmitted to the child (*see* **221 & 222**). The marked exophthalmos displays the *Stellwag sign* (*retraction of the upper eyelid*).

402

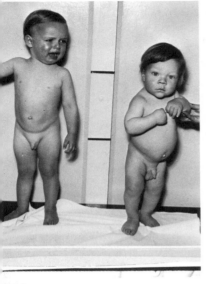

403

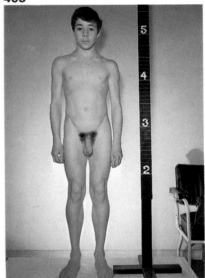

404

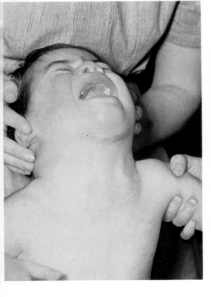

405

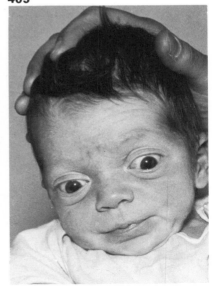

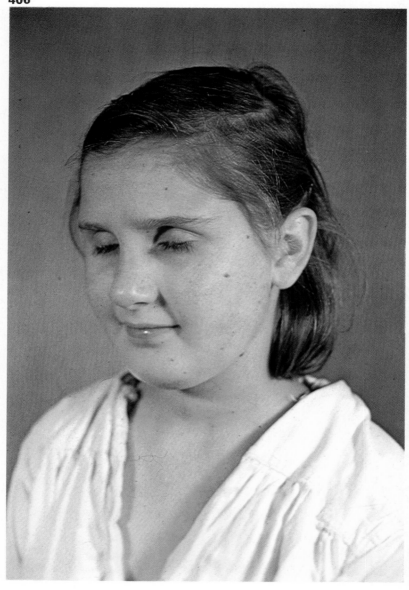

THE ADRENAL GLANDS

406 & 407 Hypoadrenalism (Addison's disease, primary adrenal hypoplasia) The 13-year-old girl was admitted in an adrenal crisis triggered off by an infection. Seen after recovery. Note the bronze pigment of the skin and the dark brown freckles on the face and chest (**406**). The pigmentation in the region of the phalangeal joints and on the finger-tips is a distinctive early sign (**407**). Tuberculosis was excluded.

407

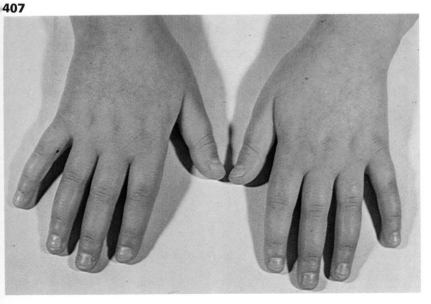

408 Hyperadrenalism (**Cushing's syndrome, adreno-cortical hyperplasia**) Exploratory surgery is indicated to exclude an adrenal or pituitary tumour. The 6-year-old girl displays *buffalo type* obesity which affects mainly the upper part of the body (*left*). Lateral view shows the accumulation of fat tissue on the back (*dowager's back*).

409 & 410 Venous insufficiency in hypercorticism is manifested by the plethoric high-coloured face and purple striae.

408

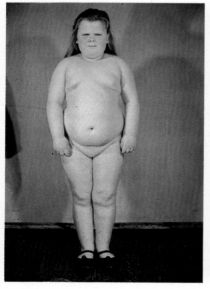
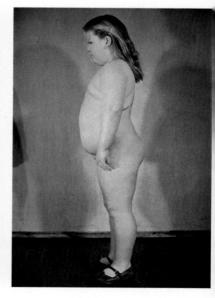

409

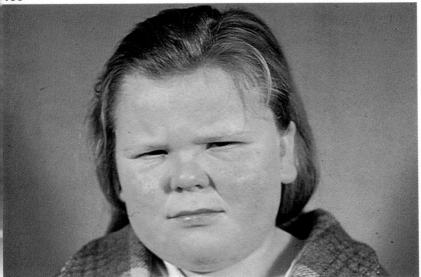

410

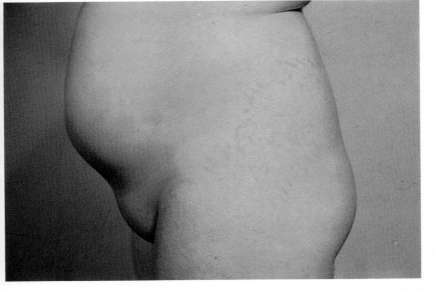

The Adreno-genital Syndrome is the result of defective cortisol synthesis. The management of these cases is confronted with difficult therapeutic and psychological problems.

411 & 412 Virilising salt-losing hyperplasia is the more common type of the syndrome, and is due to deficiency of the enzyme 21-hydroxylase. The clinical picture simulates Addison's disease or conditions with severe electrolyte disturbance. This otherwise well-developed newborn, a chromatin-positive female, displays virilisation of the external genitalia. Close-up (**412**) shows the enlarged clitoris forming a phallus, the fused, rugged labio-scrotal folds and the urogenital sinus (*see* **233 & 234**).

413 & 414 Another variant of virilisation with hypertension
Associated with 11-hydroxylase enzyme deficiency. The virilising effect is shown in an older child. This 18-month-old infant, regarded by the parents as a boy and named accordingly, is a chromatin-positive female.

Note the excessive muscular development and the accelerated growth (*Infant Hercules*). Close-up (**414**) illustrates the enlargement of the clitoris.

411

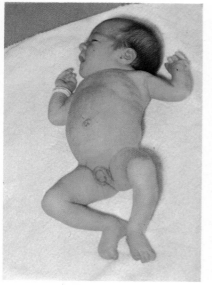

412

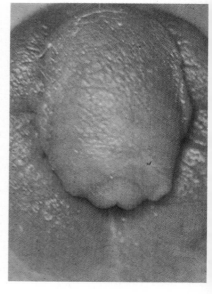

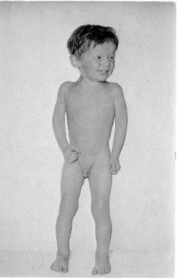
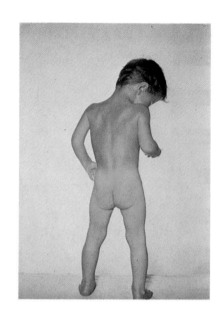

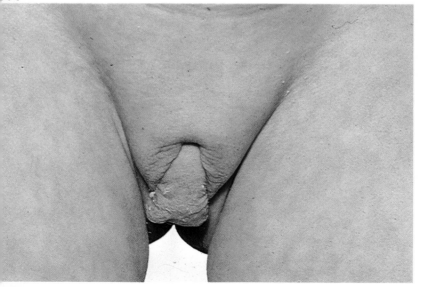

Puberty

NORMAL PUBERTY

Pubertal changes begin in girls between the ages of 10.5-11.2 years and in boys about the age of 12 years. The sequence of appearance of the pubertal phenomena varies and depends upon heredity, the hypo-thalamic-pituitary-adrenal function and the response of the end organs.

415 Normal female pubertal development Incipient breast development (*thelarche*) in a 10-year-old girl. The moderate obesity is transitory and not uncommon.

416 Same girl at 12 years The pubertal changes have progressed. There is further growth of the breasts, pigmentation of the nipples and sexual hair (*pubarche*). Menstruation (*menarche*) had started.

15

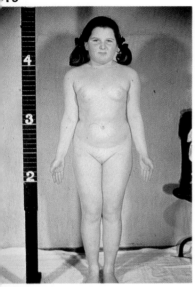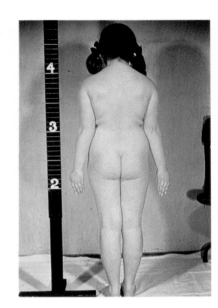

16

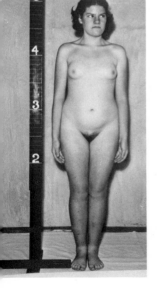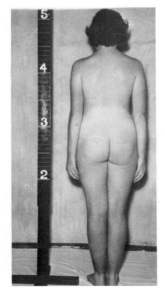

273

417

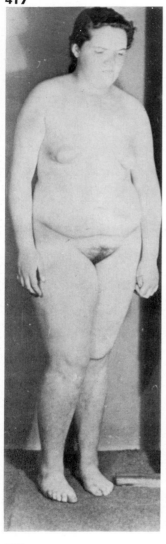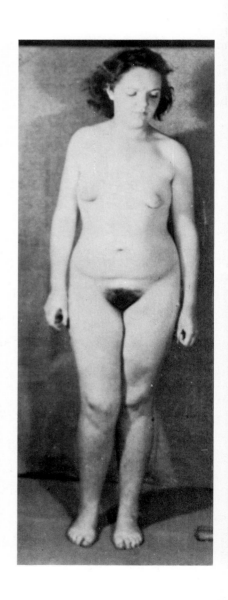

17 Striking changes may occur with maturation The un-attractive, plump girl of 10 years had grown into an attractive, well-proportioned adolescent at the age of 15½ years.

18 Normal male pubertal development The 13-year-old boy shows sexual hair and penial, testicular and scrotal growth. The moderate obesity is transitory.

18

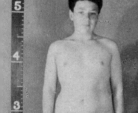
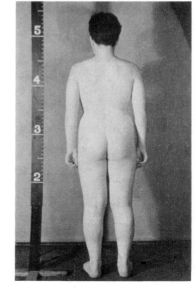

PRECOCIOUS PUBERTY

Puberty is regarded as precocious if pubertal changes appear before the age of 8.4 years in girls and before the age of 10 years in boys. Partial precocity is usually harmless and gradually changes into normal maturation. Total precocity involving all elements demands the identification of any underlying organic cause.

419 Premature breast development started in this girl at the age of 2 years. Note the different size of the breasts, observed also in normal thelarche. The condition is usually benign, but persists till puberty. No other signs of precocity were found.

420 Gynaecomastia in a 10-year-old boy. In the majority of cases this increase of glandular tissue is a transitory anomaly with spontaneous regression. Differentiate from simple adiposity.

421 Premature pubarche A precocious 7-year-old girl is seen in comparison with a normal 7-year-old. Here the presence of a brain lesion (*craniopharyngeoma*) had to be excluded. Note the stunted growth of the patient.

422 Pseudo-precocity in a 9-year-old boy with penial enlargement and pubic hair was the side-effect of medication with methyltestosterone for retarded growth. The signs regressed after withdrawal of the drug.

19

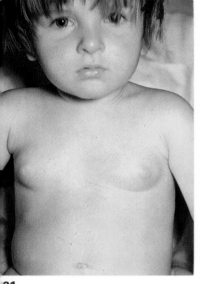

420

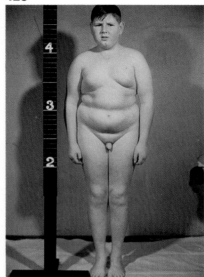

21

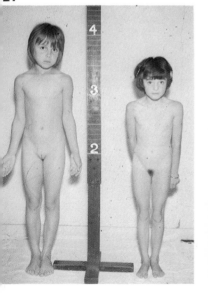

422

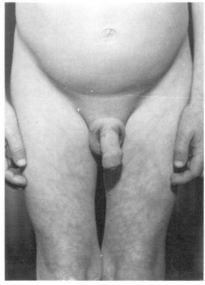

423 Precocious virilisation in a 4-year-old boy, caused by an *adreno cortical tumour.* The sexual development is consistent with an age of 12 years. Note the accelerated growth, pubic and axillary hair, and large penis. The lateral view depicts the abdominal distension due to the tumour.

424 Close-up illustrates the enlarged phallus and the pubic hair without testicular and scrotal enlargement.

425 An encapsulated carcinoma was removed Scattered smaller tumours were found in the abdomen and metastases in the regional lymphnodes.

423

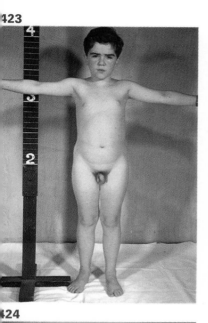

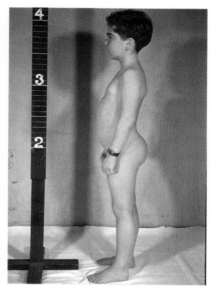

424

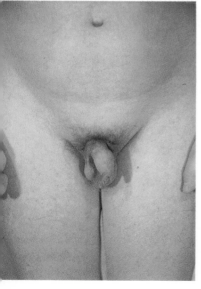

425

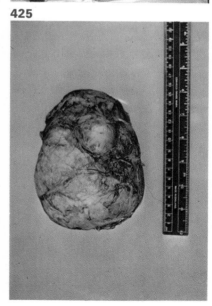

426 Precocious feminisation A *granulosa cell tumour of the ovaries* was the activating agent. The 8-year-old child shows advanced pubertal changes, hirsutes and abdominal distension. Urinary excretion of oestrogens was greatly increased.

427 The clitoris is of adult size After removal of the tumour the signs gradually regressed.

426

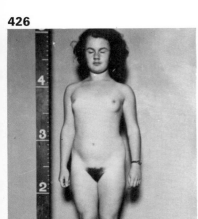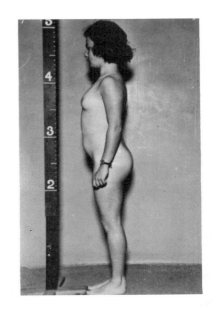

427

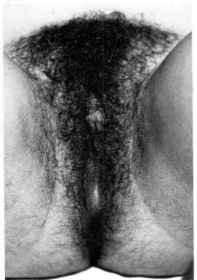

428

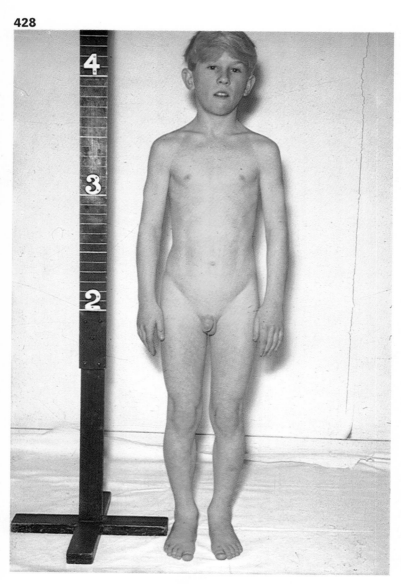

DELAYED PUBERTY

This is consistent with the failure of breast development in girls of 13 years and of genital development and growth of pubic hair in boys of 14 years. Gonadal dysgenesis has to be excluded.

428 Simple idiopathic delay of hormonal activity The development, bone age and weight of the 14-year-old boy corresponded to an age of 12 years. Note the feminine appearance. Pubertal signs appeared only at the age of 16 years.

429 & 430 Endocrine disturbance The 15-year-old girl was undersized. Note the dull expression and enlarged circumference of the neck. Biochemical investigations revealed hypothyroid values. Pubertal signs appeared with the application of replacement therapy (puberty is more often advanced in these cases).

429

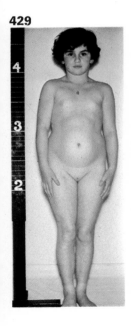 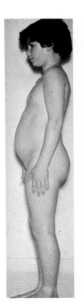

430

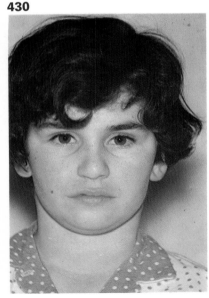

Special Syndromes

CHROMOSOME DISORDERS

Chromosome analysis of genetic disorders can correlate certain clinical signs with specific chromosome aberrations. The clinical picture is not always well-defined and signs may overlap and may even appear in individuals with a normal chromosome pattern.

Some phenotypes of more common disorders of this nature are demonstrated.

AUTOSOMAL TRISOMY

This disorder is connected with multiple anomalies, mental retardation and a high mortality rate.

Trisomy 13-15 D1 (Patau) (431-438)

431 Frontal view Note the narrow palpebral fissure, microphthalmia, depressed nasal saddle, thick nose, high philtrum, thin lips and short neck in the newborn female.

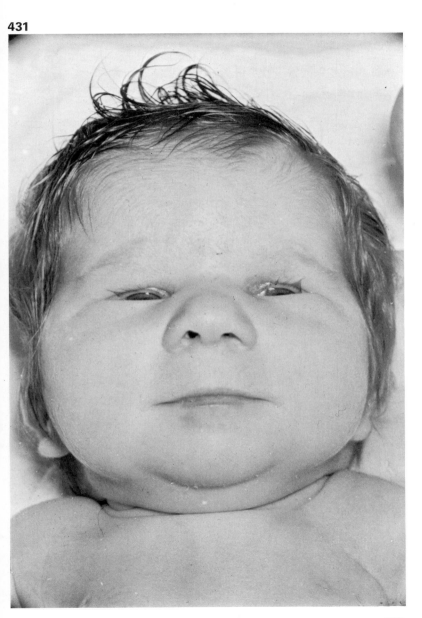

432 Lateral view shows the deformity of the low-set ears and the typical flexion and overlapping of the fingers.

433 Close-up reveals a single palmar crease (*Simian line*).

434 Polydactily There is a large first and additional sixth toe (*bottom*). Plantar flexion of the other toes is usually present. The infant was deaf.

432

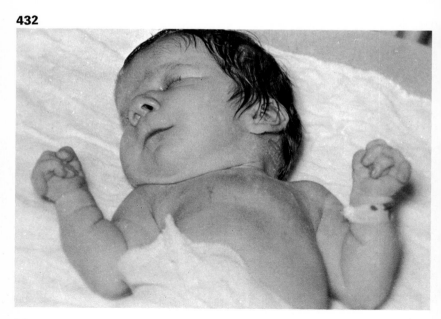

433

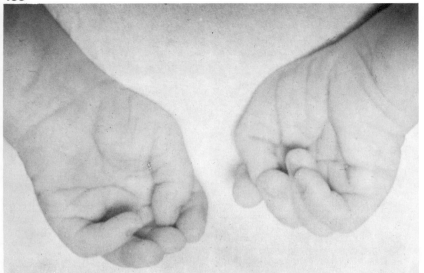

434

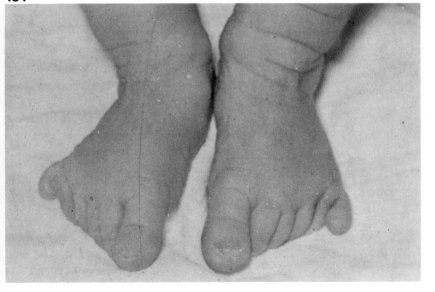

435 & 436 Variant of 13-15 D1 trisomy Additionally, the newborn female has signs of the oculo-auriculovertebral (*Goldenhar's*) syndrome. There are bilateral, fleshy *preauricular fibromas*, a low hair-line and low-set, peculiarly formed ears.

437 Close up of the face shows a total cleft of the lips, a deformed nose, hypotelorism and left-sided *anophthalmia*.

438 The same baby at 5 months after removal of the fibromas. The developmental improvement of the features is considerable.

435

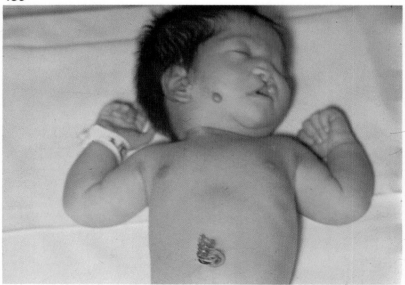

436

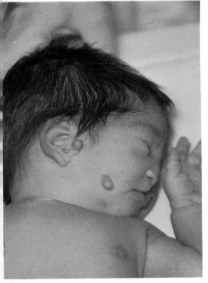

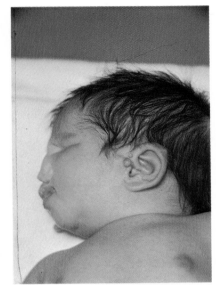

437

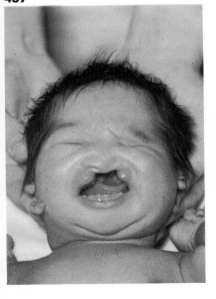

438

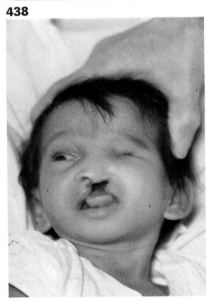

439 Trisomy 18 E1 (Edwards) Newborn female with micrognathia, low-set ears and peculiar flexion deformity of the fingers of the left hand. Arhinencephaly (*developmental arrest of the forebrain*) occurs with this syndrome.

440 A newborn with similar flexion of the fingers and bilateral Simian palmar creases. The chromosome pattern was normal. Chromosome analysis is essential in doubtful cases.

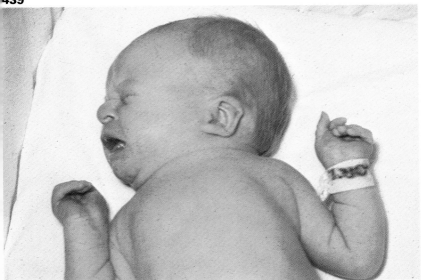

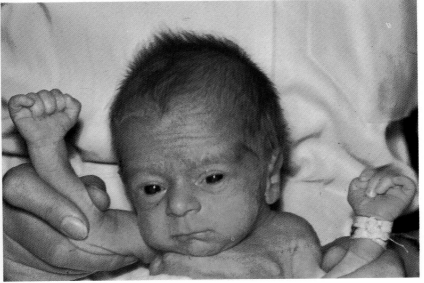

441 'Cat-cry' syndrome (Maladie du cri du chat) The features
are conspicuous ; the face is oval and the skull microcephalic. There is
hypertelorism, an antimongolian slant of the palpebral fissures, a plump
nose, high philtrum, a small mouth and low-set large ears. The cry is
high-pitched *mewing*. Deletion of the short arm of chromosome − 5 is
the usual pattern.

441

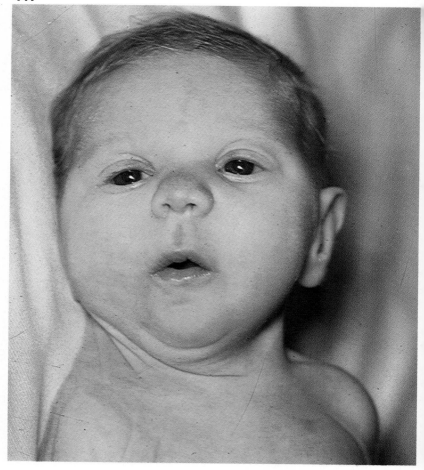

DOWN'S SYNDROME (MONGOLISM)

This is the most frequent form of chromosome deviation (1:700 live births). There are three types of this syndrome which carry different recurrence risk, which is important for genetic counselling.

It appears either as *Trisomy 21*, the regular Down's syndrome, with 47 chromosomes (95%) or as *Translocation* D/21 or G/21 with 46 chromosomes inherited from a maternal carrier, balanced or sporadic (see relevant non-related karyotypes on pages 312 and 314). *Mosaics* which are less severely affected show a mixture of normal and trisomic cells. The phenotype is basically identical. All cases are mentally retarded, but of variable severity.

The correlation of the incidence of Down's syndrome and advanced maternal age is well documented. The risk rises steeply after the age of 35 years. Chromosomal analysis of cultured foetal cells obtained by amniocentesis within the 16–18th week of gestation will establish the antenatal diagnosis and the essential karyotype.

A decision on the termination of pregnancy has to be balanced against the rearing of a disabled child needing a lifelong sheltered existence.

The stigmata are demonstrated in the following series:

442 & 443 Typical appearance of a newborn mongol Note the floppy, hypotonic posture, small round head, the slanting palpebral fissures, abdominal distension and umbilical hernia.

442

443

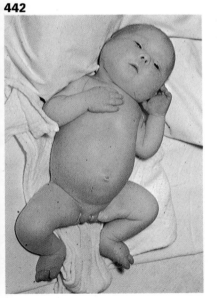 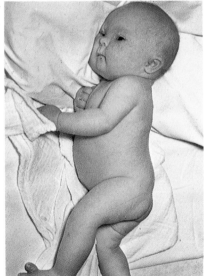

444 Low-set ears and malformed pinnae Note the flattened upper helix and preauricular sinus.

445 Another variant is the coarse broad helix and incomplete gyration.

446 Common facial features Bilateral epicanthus, a skinfold covering the medial angle of the eye, the finely drawn eyebrows, depressed nasal bridge, flaring nostrils, high-coloured cheeks and thick lips.

447 Brushfield's spots are aggregates of stromal fibres which form a ring around the iris near the limbus, and tend to disappear with age.

444

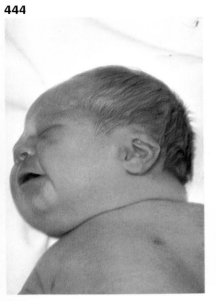

445

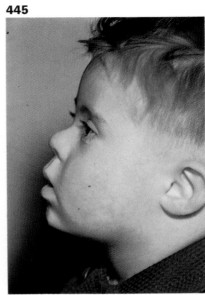

446

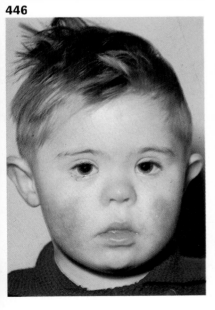

447

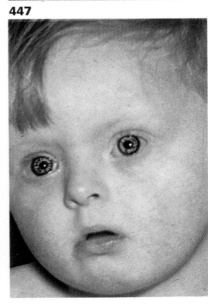

448 & 449 A high arched, narrow palate and irregular dentition
The lateral upper incisors are missing, the canini are conical. Note the gap
between the lower medial incisors.

**450 & 451 Broad, spade-like hands and abnormal dermato-
glyphics** The fingers are short and of nearly equal length (**450**). Note
the single palmar crease (*Simian line*) and the high axial triradius (**451**).

448

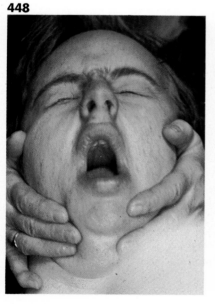

449

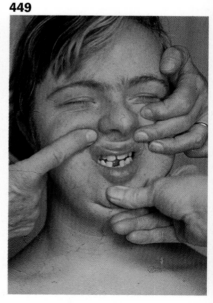

450

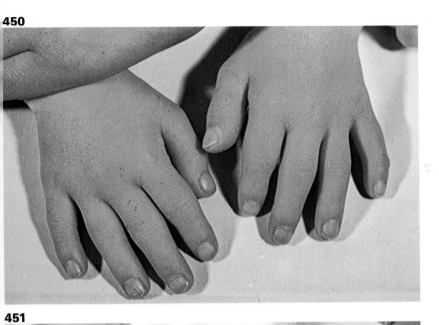

451

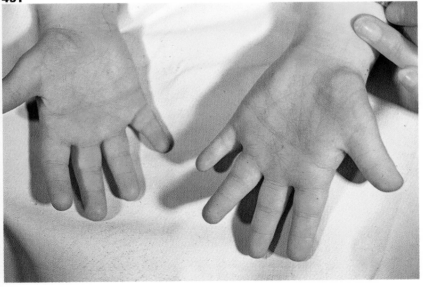

452-455 Other variants are a bridged palmar line (*Sydney line*) which becomes confluent on bending and continues towards the ulnar edge (*arrowed*) of the palm (**452**), an irregularly creased palm (**453**), a low-set thumb, a missing second joint line (**454**) and clinodactily of digit V (**455**).

452

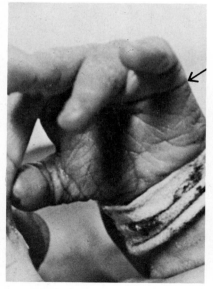

453

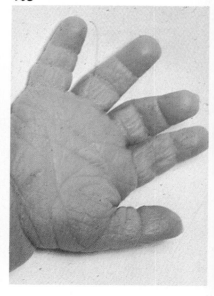

454

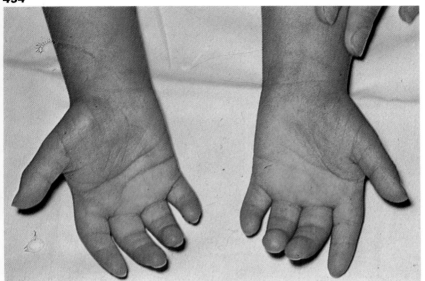

455

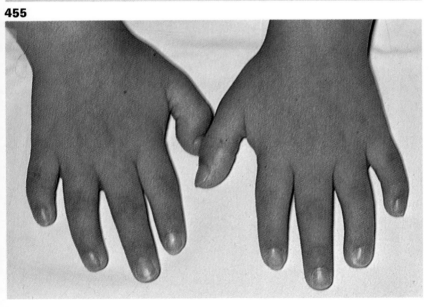

299

456 & 457 The feet are broad and short A gap exists between the first and second toe. The plantae are creased with a deep long furrow (*ape-line*) between the first and second toe.

456

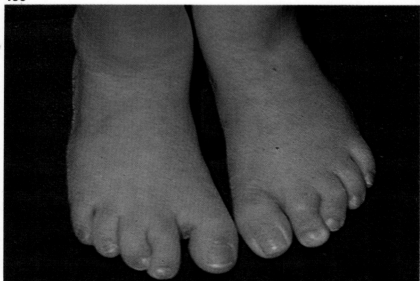

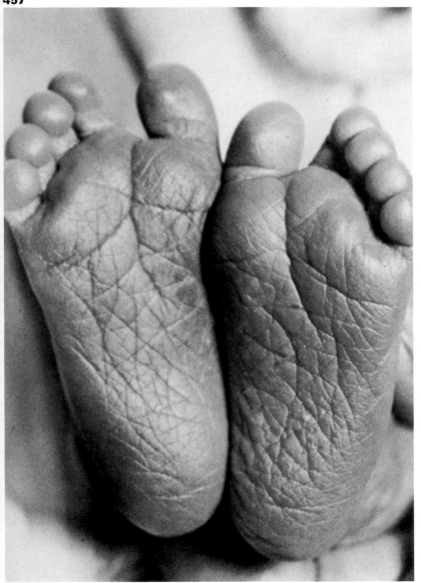

458 & 459 Muscular hypotony allows an increased range of joint movements without discomfort.

460 & 461 Development of stance is delayed The 2-year-old boy is unable to stand without help. The 3-year-old girl is standing on a wide base with adducted feet to maintain the balance.

458

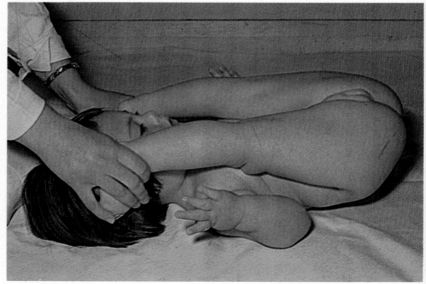

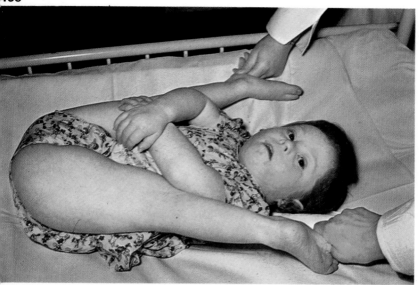

459

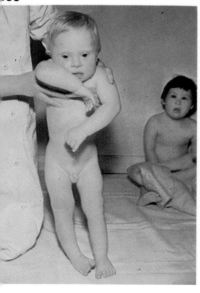

460

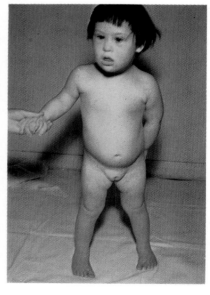

461

462 & 463 Peculiar mannerisms of movement and posture The tilting of head and body and the clasping and wringing of the hands are particularly characteristic.

The stigmata described are present in all cases, but with different degrees of expressivity, thus preserving some individuality and even family likeness. Consequently there are pitfalls in recognising cases, especially in the newborn. The diagnosis is established by chromosome analysis.

464 Newborn female Here the facial aspect is not characteristic.

465 Same baby The hypotonic posture and 'frog-like' position are suspicious.

462

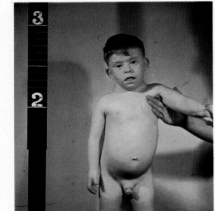
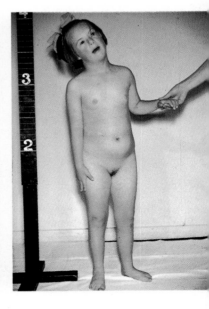

463

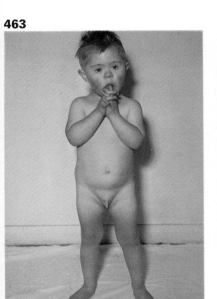

464

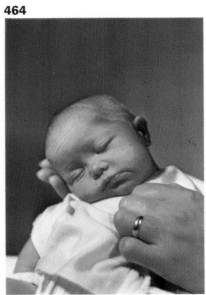

465

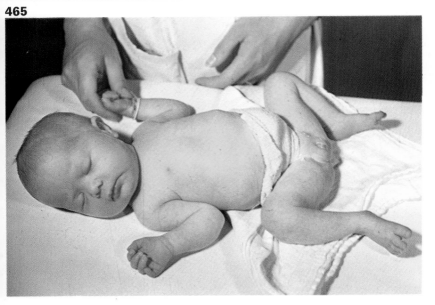

466 A 7-day-old female The puffy face and protruding tongue may resemble hypothyroidism (*left*). Crying makes the condition more obvious (*right*).

467 A spot diagnosis can be misleading The facial features are peculiar. One of these babies is a cretin, one a mosaic and one a mongol. Can you diagnose them correctly? (*answer at top overleaf*).

466

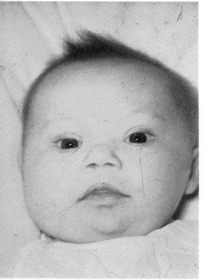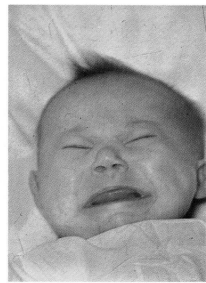

467

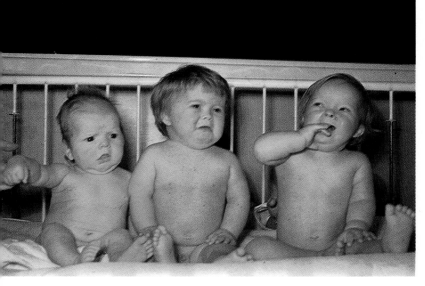

468-473 Features of the older child vary from a near normal appearance to obvious abnormality. Study the facial aspects of these six mongoloid children ranging from puckish, alert and interested, to open-mouthed, dull, and expressionless.

468

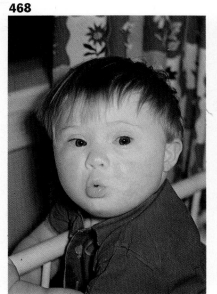

469

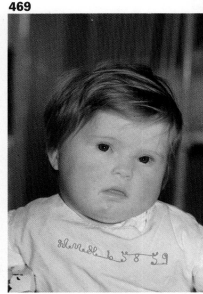

308

470

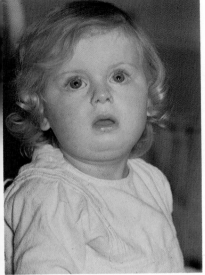

471

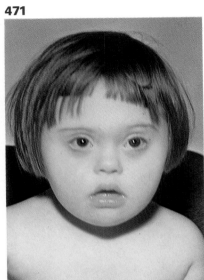

472

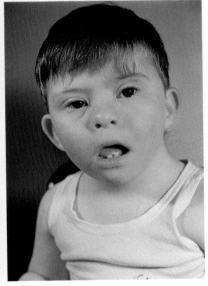

473

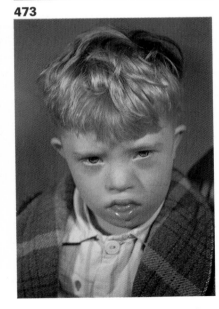

474 Family likeness A 6-year-old mongol (*left*) seen with her 5-year old sister. Note the contrast in height.

474

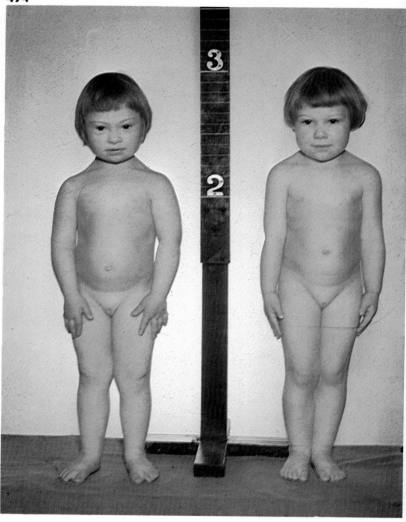

The majority of mongols are stunted, but normal growth and sexual development may occur. Few cases are educable, most are trainable for manual occupations.

475 & 476 A 'low-grade' mongol (IQ 20) 19 years old. He is of adequate physical development. The stigmata are obvious.

475

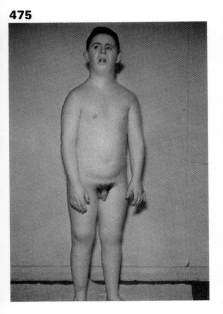

476

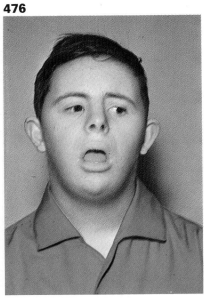

477-480 A 5-year-old mongol (IQ 45) with typical features. At the age of 17 years (**479 & 480**), growth and sexual development are normal and the mongolian features are now hardly noticeable, but the dull expression reveals the retardation.

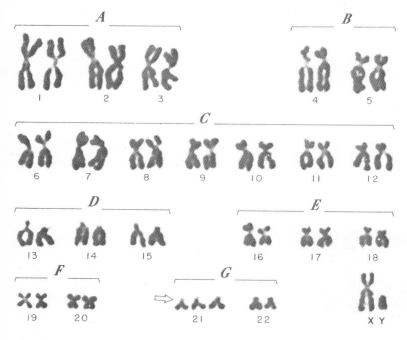

Karyotype of mongol with 21-trisomy. It has been agreed by cytogeneticists that the 'mongol chromosome' will be called chromosome 21. The patient is male, XY.
(Preparation by Dr. F. Sergovich)

477

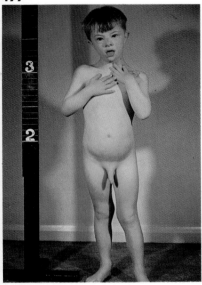

478

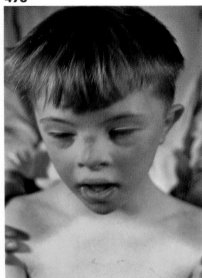

479

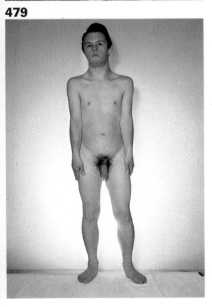

480

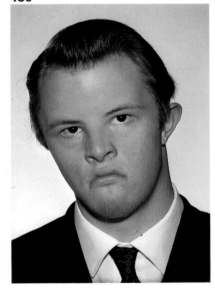

481-484 A 'high-grade' mongol (IQ 62) seen at the age of 7 and of 19 years. This obviously affected boy grew into an unobtrusive adolescent, but did not qualify for formal education.

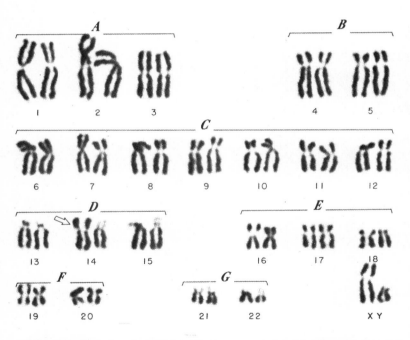

Translocation mongol. Three 21 chromosomes are present, but one has become translocated on to a 14 chromosome. This can happen (as in this case) as a 'de novo' event or it can happen as the result of an inherited translocation.
(Preparation by Dr. F. Sergovich)

481

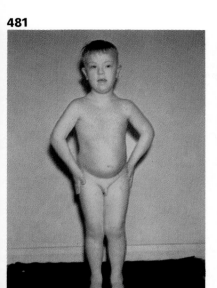

482

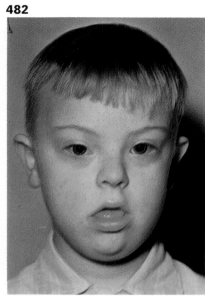

483

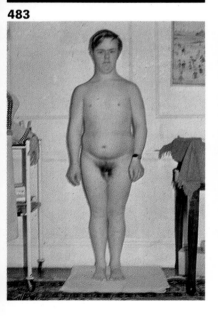

484

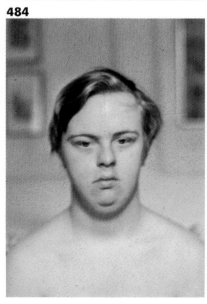

MENTAL DEFICIENCY

A disorder resulting from various causes, congenital or acquired, which prevents normal brain development. The affected child is unable to achieve social independence and needs special training and custodial care for life.

485 Brain damage A 3-year-old child acting on the level of a 6-month-old. The *setting sun* sign indicates brain dysfunction (*see* **250**).

486 Severely retarded 2-year-old The condition followed a forceps delivery. Note the infantile posture. Masturbation was persistent and compulsive.

485

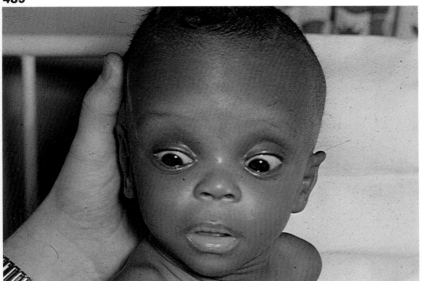

486

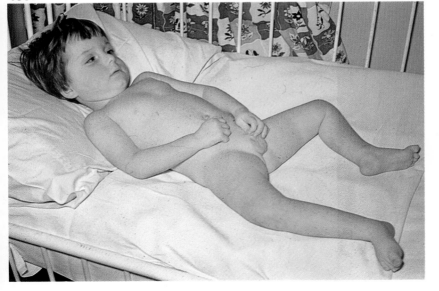

487 Primary amentia The 3-year-old girl is physically well-developed. Behaviour is hyperkinetic. Expression and attitude reveal her mental retardation.

488 Oligophrenia in an 18-month-old boy. Milestones were retarded. He has a short neck, but no other anomalies.

489 Same child at 8 years of age had developed adiposo-genital dystrophy and marked genua valga. Mental retardation was severe.

487

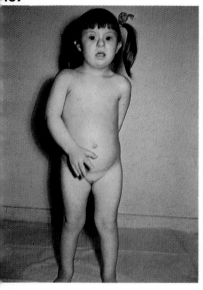

488

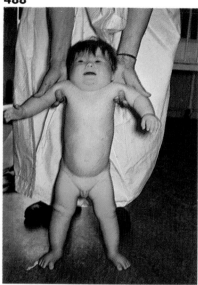

489

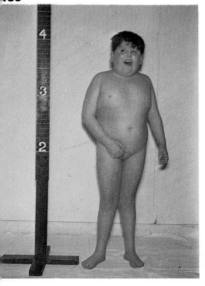

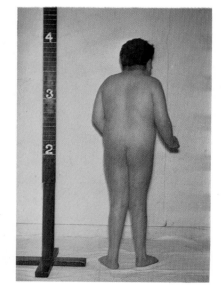

INFANTILE AUTISM

This severe emotional disorder, emanating from a disturbed mother-child relationship, usually develops before the age of 3 years. The behaviour is marked by obsessive loneness, lack of speech and attachment to persons, reiterative purposeless movements and outbreaks of severe temper tantrums.

Generally these children are not mentally retarded but may become psychotic.

490-492 Autistic behaviour Note the infantile posture and detachment of this $2\frac{1}{2}$-year-old child. She had a peculiar affinity to round objects which were twisted and turned without purpose. When approached she turns away, withdrawn, thumbsucking.

490

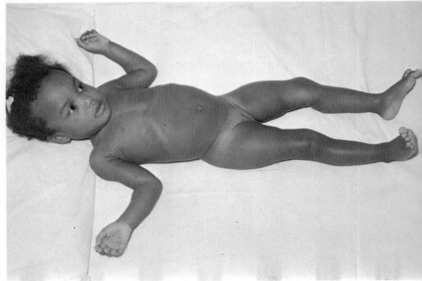

491

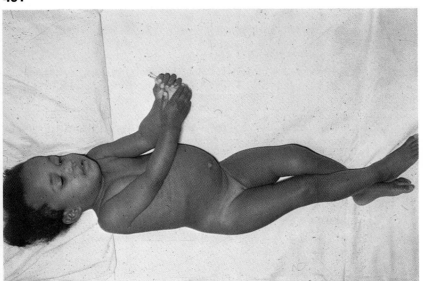

492

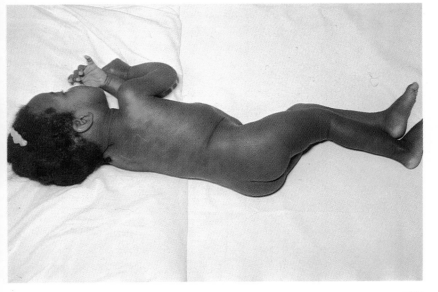

SKELETAL DYSPLASIAS

These are genetic disorders leading to a strikingly bizarre appearance and dwarfing. The signs are often overlapping, but the different pathogenesis establishes these disorders as independent entities. Advance in biochemical investigations has succeeded in correlating some of these conditions with inborn errors of metabolism consisting of specific enzyme defects.

493 Achondroplasia (chondrodystrophy, rhizomatic dwarfism) is the result of defective endochondral growth and ossification. This 15-month-old dwarf shows the distinctive disproportionate build of a large square head, a normally-sized, laterally compressed trunk and short proximal parts of arms and legs (*rhizomelic micromelia*).

The lateral view depicts the bossing forehead, depressed nasal saddle, marked lordosis and spade-like hand (*trident hand*).

494 Same child at 3 years has grown to only half the size of a normal child (*sitting height is normal*).

493

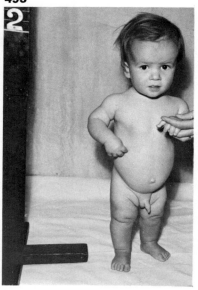
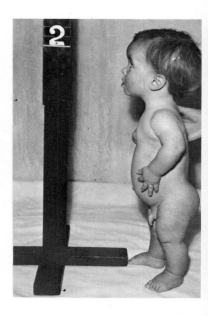

494

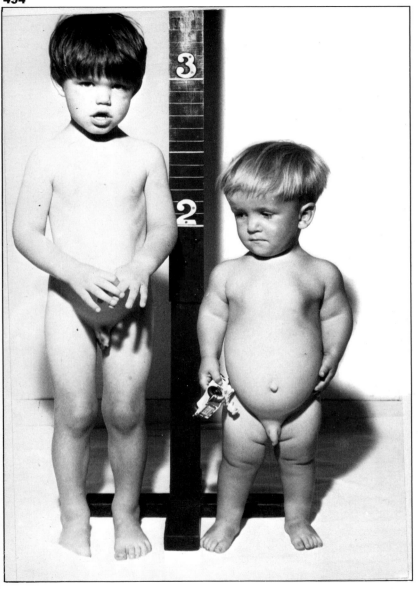

495 X-ray of the skull shows its large size, the shortened base and shallow sella turcica, signs characteristic of this dysplasia.

496 & 497 The bones are broad and short The epiphyseal lines are irregular and flared ; the metacarpal bones show some cupping.

498 Pseudo-achondroplasia (hypochondroplasia) The 5-year-old dwarfed girl has some features resembling achondroplasia. Head and arms are of normal size, but the legs are short.

495

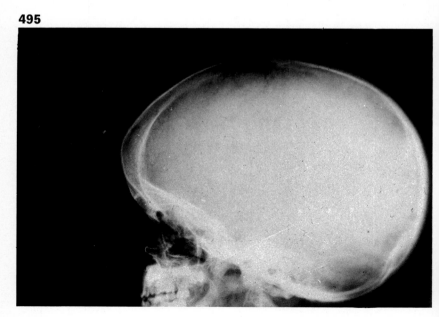

496

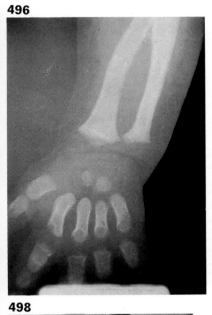

497

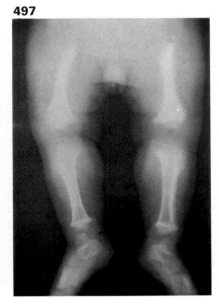

498

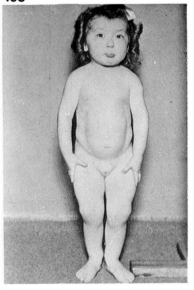
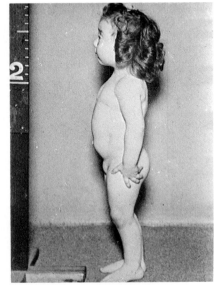

499 & 500 Thanatophoric dwarfism A severe deformity with large head and micromelia, often diagnosed as achondroplasia. X-ray shows severely distorted bones, cupping of the epiphyseal lines, osteoporosis and multiple fracture lines resembling osteogenesis imperfecta (Lobstein's disease) or hypophosphataemia. These children do not survive.

The condition is of autosomal recessive inheritance. Antenatal diagnosis by ultrasonic measurements of the foetal limbs at the 16th week of gestation or by foetoscopy is indicated in cases of risk.

Mucopolysaccharidoses (501-506) are autosomal recessive inherited disorders of the mucopolysaccharide metabolism due to deficiency of specific lysosomal hydrolase activity. The storage of faulty metabolites may lead to severe bone dysplasias, dwarfism, visceromegaly, corneal clouding, vascular and cardiac degeneration, and mental retardation. Large amounts of abnormal acid mucopolysaccharides (*glycosaminoglycans*) are found in the urine and metachromatic granules in white blood cells and in cultured fibroblasts. Antenatally the condition is detectable by the metachromasia of amniotic cells.

So far six genetically and biochemically distinct disorders have been differentiated.

501 & 502 Dysostosis multiplex (Hurler's disease, Mucopolysaccharidosis 1) is the most common form. The ugly, coarse features resembling a *gargoyle*, and the hypertrichosis in this 2-year-old child are characteristic. X-ray of the skeleton will show hook-shaped deformity of the first lumbar vertebrae forming a *gibbus*, and distortion of the epiphyseal ends of the long bones. The child was blind, deaf and mentally retarded.

499

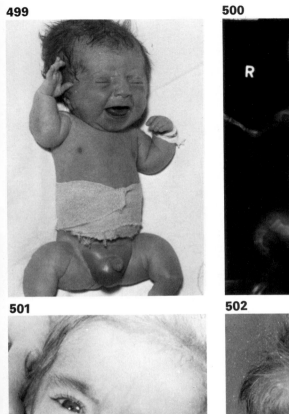

500

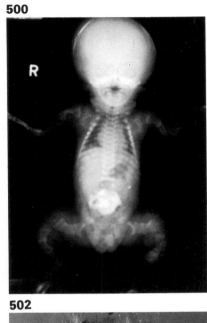

R

501

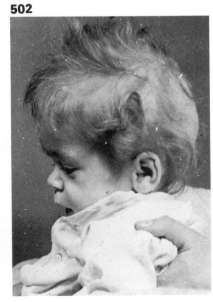

502

503-506 Spondylo-epiphyseal dysplasia (Morquio's disease, mucopolysaccharidosis IV) This variant is shown at the age of 2 days and of 18 months. In the newborn the ugly features, coarse, broad hands and distorted, knobbly contures of the limbs are suggestive of the disorder. At the age of 18 months the baby had grown into a grotesque, disproportionate dwarf (**504**). Note the large head, protruding chin, the short neck and trunk, and pigeon chest. The lateral view shows the marked iordosis and the short, deformed limbs fixed in semi-flexion (**505**). The child cannot lie flat (**506**). Corneal clouding, aortic regurgitation, mental impairment and keratosulfaturia were further characteristic features.

The remaining syndromes in this group are: Hunter's II Sanfillipo's III, Scheie's V and Maroteaux-Lamy's VI. They differ in severity of connective tissue involvement, physical deformities and mental retardation, and the type of acid mucopolysaccharides stored and excreted in the urine.

(*For other inborn errors of metabolism see* **282-285, 411-414**.)

503

504

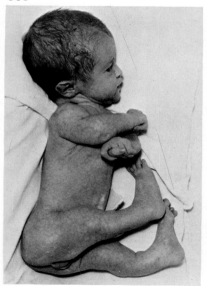

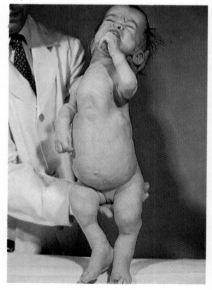

505

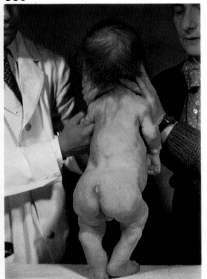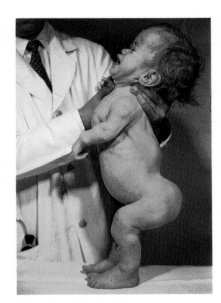

506

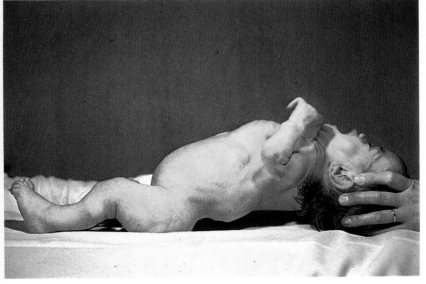

329

507-510 An 'odd looking' child with micromelia This baby shows a peculiar combination of achondroplastic and spondylo-epiphyseal features. The large head, the attractive intelligent face and the normally sized trunk are in contrast with the marked gibbus, stiff, very short limbs and the contracture of the hip joints limiting the upright stance.

The urine was free of abnormal metabolites. The x-ray of the skeleton was inconclusive.

507

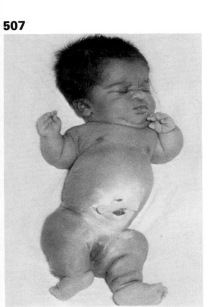

508

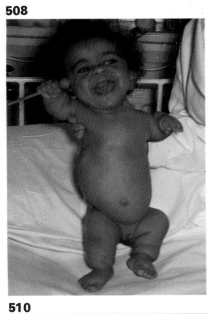

509

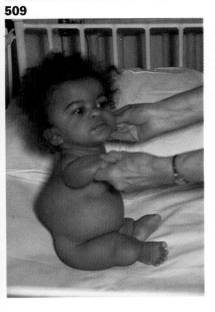

510

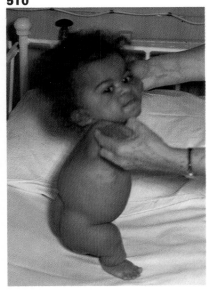

511 Osteopetrosis, marble bones (Albers-Schönberg's disease) appears in malignant form in infants and in a more benign form in later childhood. The former is illustrated. This 4-day-old baby was deaf and blind. The femur fractured during delivery. Note the large head, leftsided ptosis, necrotic pressure mark on the right deltoid region and paralysis of the legs.

512 X-ray shows the dense sclerotic bones, a fractured femur and a large liver shadow. The baby died at the age of 3 months.

513 Autopsy revealed hydrocephalus, hepatosplenomegaly and gross atrophy of the brain with cyst formation.

511

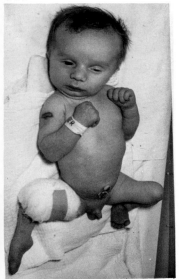

512

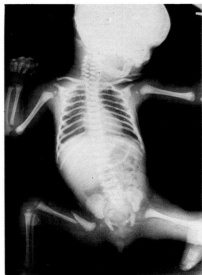

513

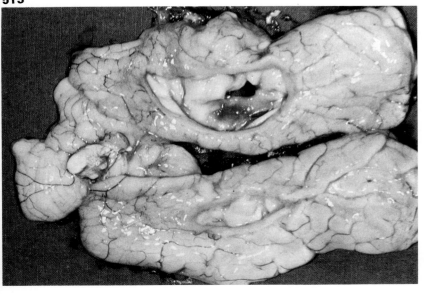

514 Klippel-Feil syndrome (congenital brevicollis) Fusion or malformation of the cervical and upper thoracic vertebrae produces the short neck and limitation of movements often associated with other skeletal and cardiovascular lesions. The hair is kept long for cosmetic reasons.

515 Cleidocranial dysostosis Aplasia or defective development of the claviculae and laxity of the ligaments allows the forward folding of the shoulders. Defective mineralization of other parts of the skeleton may occur.

514

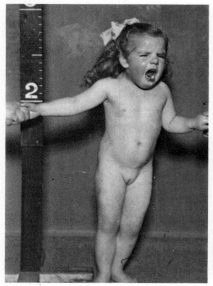
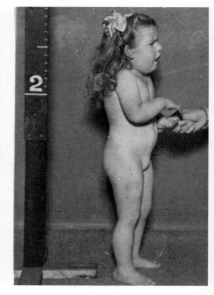

515

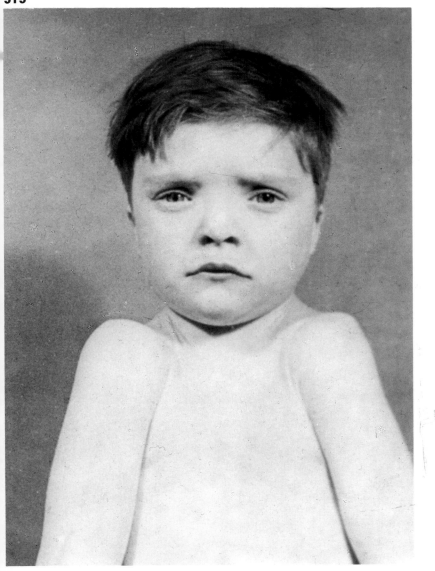

516 Acrocephalo-syndactily (Apert's syndrome) in a newborn girl. A condition of sporadic occurrence. Acrocephaly, syndactily of fingers and toes and a cleft palate are the principal signs. Cranial stenosis will cause blindness and mental retardation.

517-519 Close-up shows the antimongolian slant of the eyes, low-set, large ears, fleshy tongue, a short frenulum and the lack of hand and foot segmentation.

516

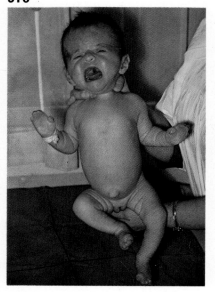

517

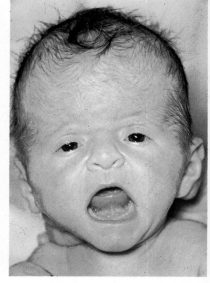

518

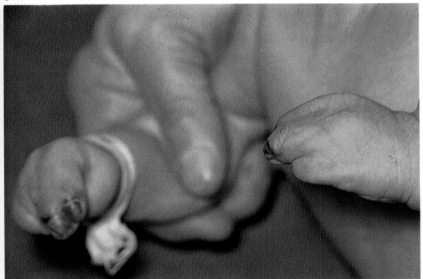

519

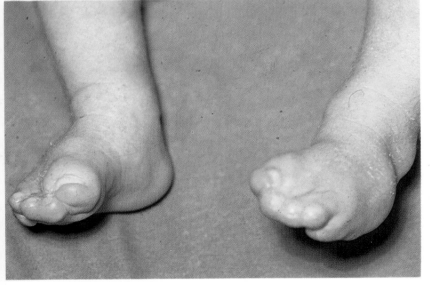

337

Craniofacial dysostosis (Crouzon's disease) (520-527) An auto-somal dominant condition characterized by early simultaneous synostosis of the coronal, sagittal and metopic sutures, resulting in progressive cranial stenosis and hypoplasia of the facial bones.

520 & 521 Appearance at birth is not distinctive, apart from hyper-telorism and a high forehead.

522-524 At 3 months the peculiar physiognomy and acrocephaly have developed. The engorged vessels indicate intracranial hypertension.

520

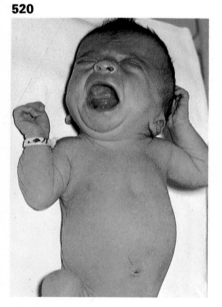

521

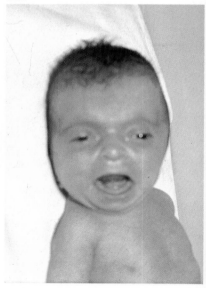

522

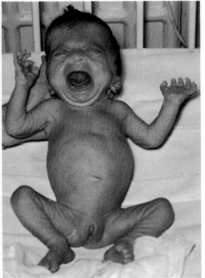

523

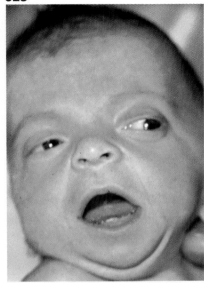

524

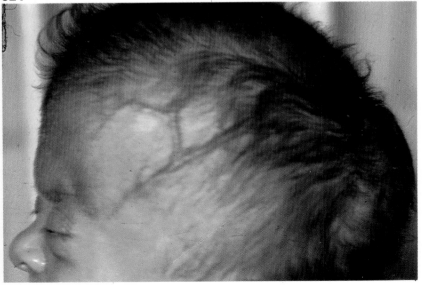

525 & 526 At 6 months the general condition has deteriorated (*cerebral dystrophy*). The face is asymmetric and flat. Antimongolian slant, exophthalmos and a divergent pseudo-strabism have developed.

527 Another peculiarity is the prominence of the central ridge on the hard palate. Craniectomy was performed later.

525

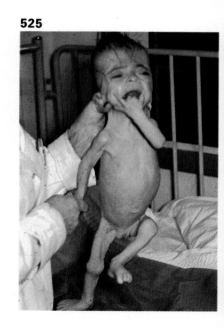

526

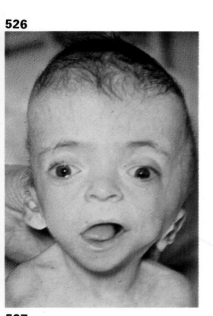
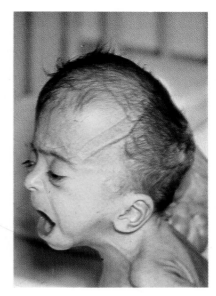

527

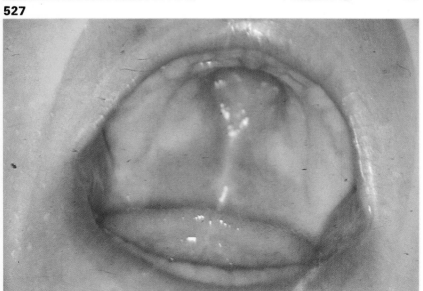

Mandibulofacial dysostosis (Treacher-Collins-Franceschetti syndrome) (528-531) A hereditary familial malformation involving the structures originating from the 1st branchial arch. Formation of face and ears is mainly affected. Variable degrees of deafness are present.

528 Appearance at birth Note the hypotrophic body and the *fish-like* physiognomy.

529 Close-up of the face shows the antimongolian slant, notching of the lateral part of the lower eyelids, deficient eyelashes, hypoplasia of the zygomatic bones and micrognathia.

530 Lateral view of malformed auricles Meatal atresia was also present.

531 Cleft of the soft palate and uvula.

528

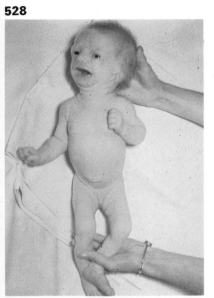

529

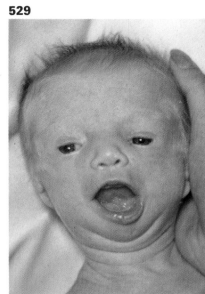

530

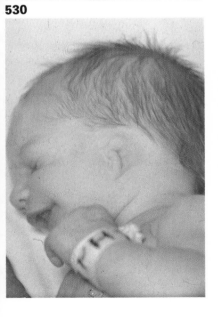

531

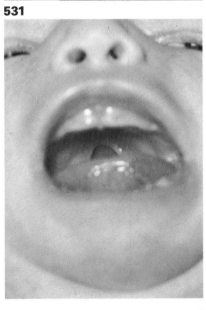

532 & 533 Another case of moderate expressivity Newborn of similar physiognomy without ear deformity.

534 Dyscephaly (Hallerman-Streiff-Francois syndrome) A craniofacial dysplasia with eye defects and skeletal and other anomalies. The head and face are *bird-like* with a beaked nose, microphthalmia, antimongolian slant and micrognathia, particularly alveolar hypoplasia. The mother showed similar features.

532

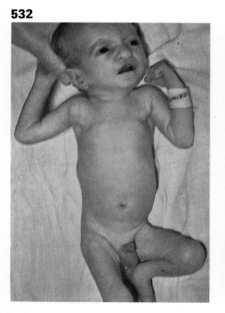

533

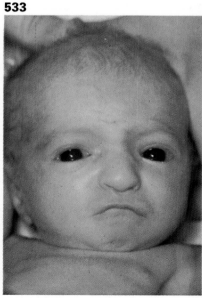

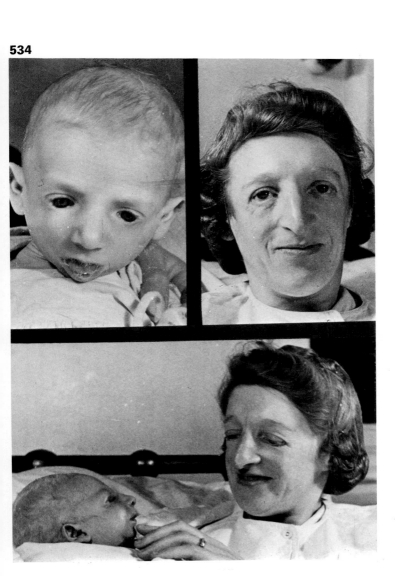

535 Typus degenerativus amstelodamensis (Cornelia de Lange-Brachman syndrome) A complex anomaly, seen in a 15-month-old girl; birthweight 1405g. Her appearance was typical; small stature, short neck, limited extension in the elbow joints, small hands and feet, flexion deformity of the fingers.

536 Close-up shows the bushy hair, low hairline, confluent thick eyebrows (*synophrys*), short nose with upturned nostrils, long philtrum, thin upper lip curving downwards (*carp mouth*), low-set ears. The expression is mask-like. These children are mentally retarded.

535

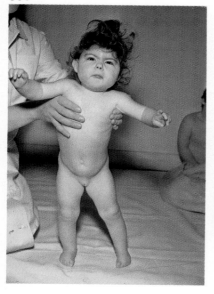

536

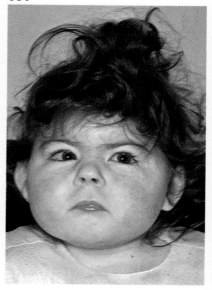

Medianfacial defects and holoprosencephaly (537-546) are seen in graded severity.

537 The mildest form This newborn has ocular hypotelorism, hypoplasia of the facial bones, redundant facial skin and a plump, broad nose. The condition becomes more obvious when crying.

537

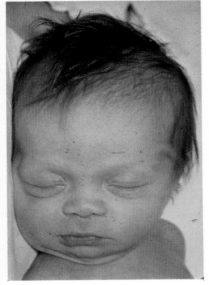
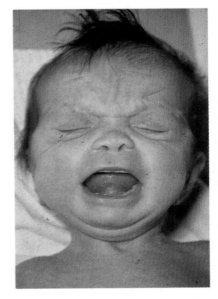

538 Another variant The baby has hypotelorism, a flat nasal saddle, a deformed nose and excessive skinfolds. The father had the same anomalies and a cleft lip. Note the *neonatal blenorrhoea* on the right eye.

539 Holoprosencephaly-arhinencephaly There is marked hypotelorism, a wide median total cleft, aplasia of the nasal septum and philtrum, a single nasal orifice and flaring nostrils. This phenotype is usually associated with alobar brain malformations. Survival is short.

540 Cyclopia The severest form of cerebro-facial dysplasia. The body is otherwise well-developed.

538

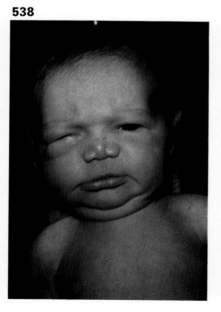

539

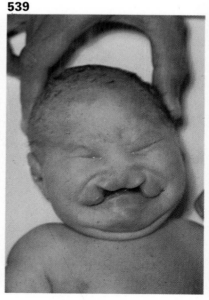

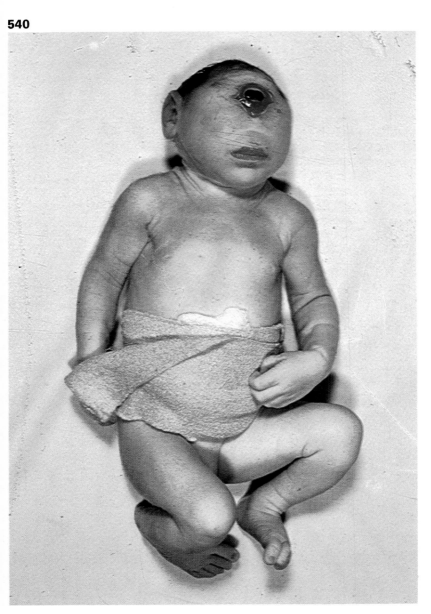

541 Close-up shows severe microcephaly, a single, large orbital cavity with fused eyeballs, a rudimentary nose set up against the long philtrum by a deep groove. The child lived for several days. Autopsy revealed fused frontal lobes and a single optic tract. Olfactory tracts were missing.

542 Pierre Robin syndrome Note the hypoplastic mandible, the severe degree of micrognathia and the malformed, flat auricle. Respiratory and feeding difficulties occur due to glossoptosis, a backward displaced tongue.

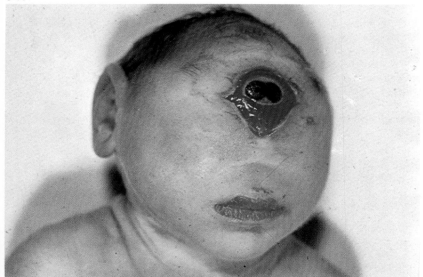

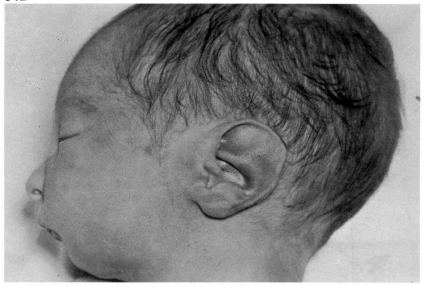

Infantile cortical hyperostosis (Caffey's syndrome) (543-546)
An acute condition of early infancy. Recently recurrence in later childhood has been reported.

543 & 544 At 3 months The well-nourished baby has marked swelling of the face localised over the jaw. The extremities are similarly affected.

545 X-ray Periosteal thickening of the long bones (*radius and ulna*) with translucent bands at the distal epiphyseal ends is diagnostic.

546 At a later stage the bones expand and the cortex is thinned. The enlarged medullary cavity has little trabeculation. The soft tissue is swollen. The condition is self-limiting.

543

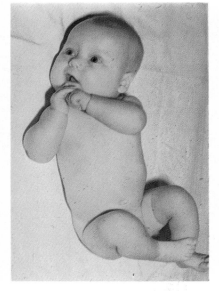

544

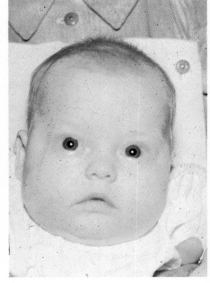

545

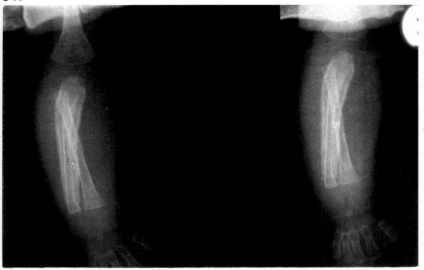

546

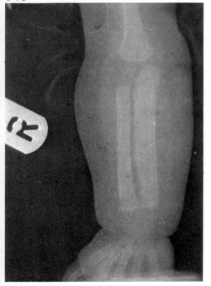

SKIN DISORDERS

Encephalotrigeminal angiomatosis (Sturge-Weber-Dimitri syndrome) (547-549)

547 Newborn with a naevus flammeus The unilateral extension from the midline along the distribution of the 1st branch of the trigeminal nerve is suggestive of intracerebral vascular abnormalities leading to brain atrophy and ocular lesions. Skull x-ray would disclose 'tramline' calcifications.

548 & 549 A similar case The lesion has progressed in this 18-month-old child. Note the blepharospasm on the left side, the bilateral buphthalmos and enlarged pupils. The intraocular pressure was raised.

547

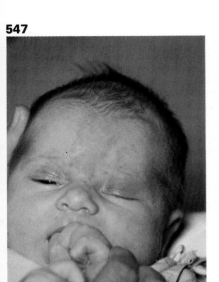

548

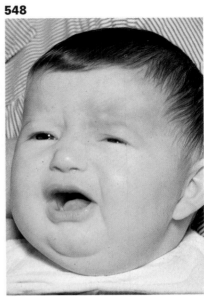

549

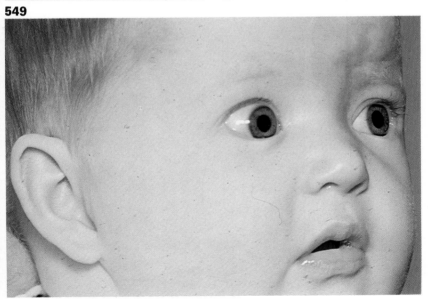

550-552 Cutis hyperelastica (Ehler-Danlos syndrome) A connective tissue disorder with hyperelastosis and reduction of collagen. The skin folds of this newborn can be pulled away from the body, even from parts where skin attachment is firm, e.g. from the hip (*dermato-chalasia*). Extreme fragility of the skin and hyperflexibility of the joints develop later.

553 Redundant cervical skin This should not be confused with hyperelastosis. The condition may be connected with chromosome aberration.

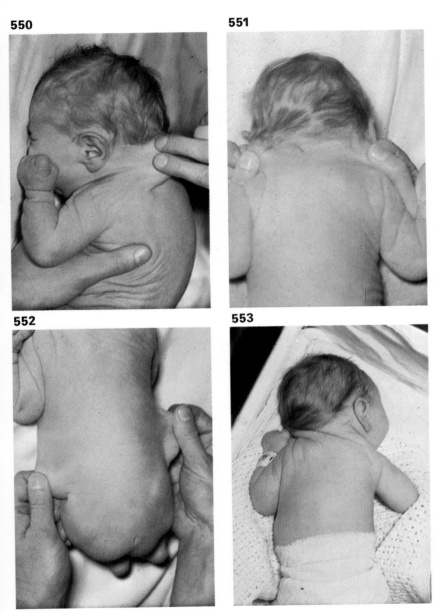

Erythema multiforme (554-557) An allergic toxic manifestation, in this case a reaction to long-acting sulfonamides.

554 Appearance The 5-month-old infant had been treated for a respiratory infection. The rash covers mainly the skin of the face, neck and trunk.

555 & 556 Close-up The different stages of the eruption are seen. There are confluent plaques on the scalp and upper parts of the face, surrounded by dark crusts. The trunk is covered with bullous lesions, some with central necrosis, surrounded by an elevated erythematous halo.

557 Cortisone treatment had a striking therapeutic effect.

554

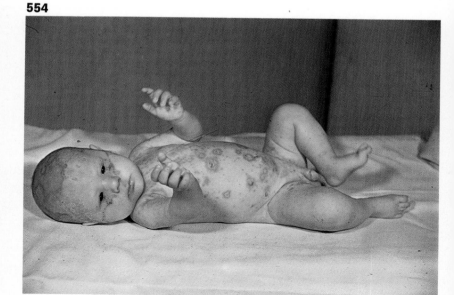

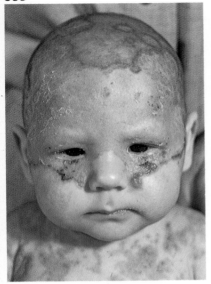

555

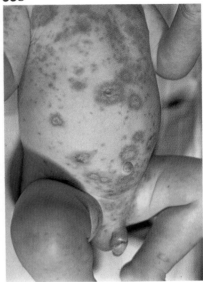

556

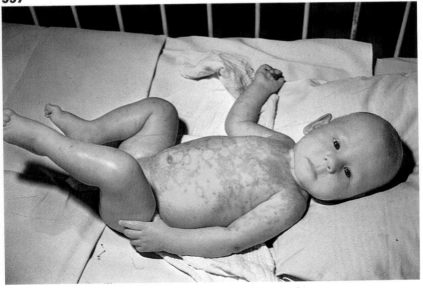

557

558 & 559 Acrodynia (Pink disease) A sensitivity reaction to prolonged intake of medicaments containing mercury (*e.g. teething powder, calomel*). Paraesthesia and extreme sweating of hands and feet induce constant rubbing and scratching and general irritability. The skin of the hands becomes sodden and peels off in large plaques (**558**). The plantae are red and oedematous (**559**). The condition is now rare as the sale of these drugs is controlled.

558

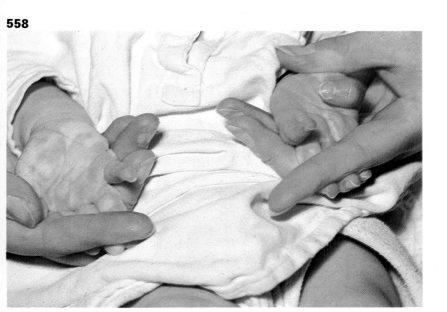

559

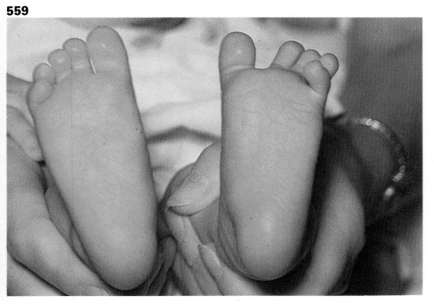

560 & 561 Neurofibromatosis (von Recklinghausen's disease)
An autosomal, dominant condition with widespread dissemination of
neurofibromas and distinctive pigmentation. Neurinomas, which occur
intracranially, involve the acoustic and optic nerve. Several members of
the family were affected. The 3-month-old infant shows brownish-red
cutaneous neurofibromas on the body and *café-au-lait* pigmentation on
the right shoulder.

560

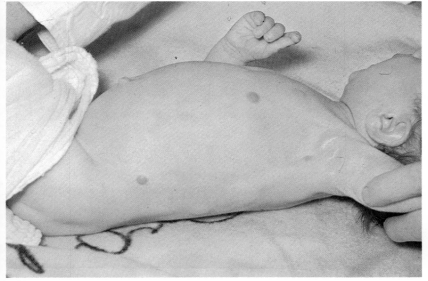

561

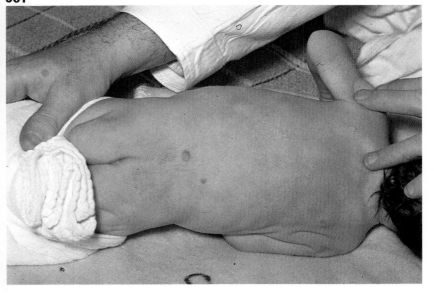

INTESTINAL AND UROGENITAL DISORDERS

**Congenital aganglionic megacolon (Hirschsprung's disease)
(562-563)** Submucosal agangliosis of the rectosigmoid leads to
dilatation and hypertrophy of the colon above the stricture, and severe
constipation. The condition is familial with male preference.

562 Distended abdomen contrasts with the poor general condition of
this 8-month-old.

563 An autopsy specimen The rectosigmoid segment is narrow and
there is hypertrophy of the proximal colon.

564 Functional megacolon Abdominal distension results from
hypotony of abdominal muscles and chronic constipation. The 2-year-
old girl has Down's syndrome.

562

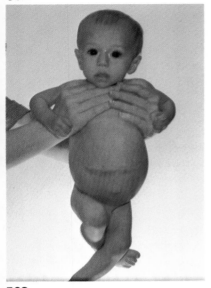
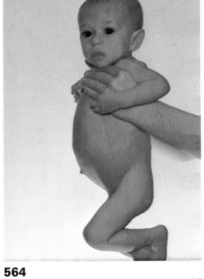

563

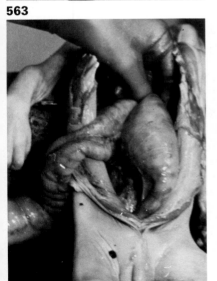

564

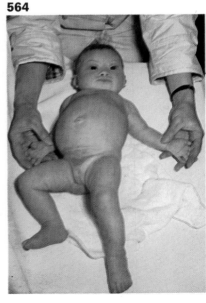

565 Obstruction by a meconium plug The newborn has abdominal distension and visible peristalsis. The condition was relieved by removal of the plug.

Megaloureter (566-569) The aetiology resembles that of Hirschsprung's disease, which often is associated. It is assumed that faulty parasympathetic innervation leads to defective detrusor function, bladder dilation and reflux. Anatomical obstruction has to be excluded.

566-568 Newborn with several peculiar features Low-set, malformed ears and heavy skinfolds under the eyes are reminiscent of *Potter's face.* He developed urinary symptoms.

569 Retrograde pyelography A dilated bladder, bilateral tortuous megaloureters and right-sided hydronephrosis were revealed.

565

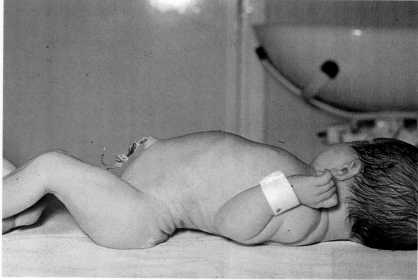

566

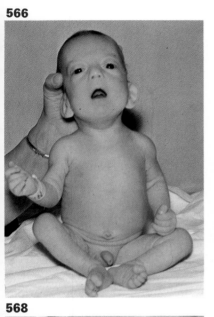

567

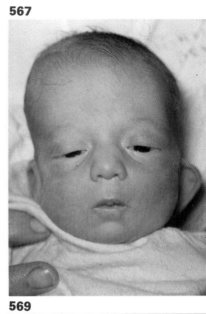

568

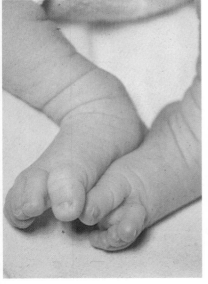

569

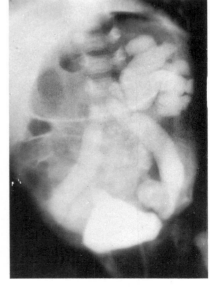

570 & 571 Renal agenesis The newborn did not have the classic Potter's face. The low-set ears were the only feature pointing to renal abnormality. Note the cleft, bifid chin, the antimongolian slant and flexure deformity of the hands resembling the Trisomy 18 E1 syndrome.

570

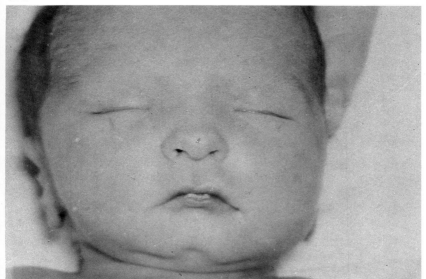

571

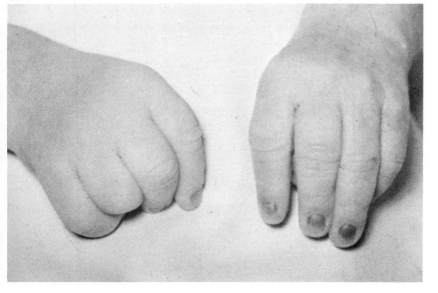

HAIR DISORDERS

Excessive hairiness (*hirsutism*) and loss of hair (*alopecia*) are associated with various disorders. Some separate entities of hair disorders are demonstrated.

572 Hypotrichosis The scalp of the newborn is sparsely covered with fine *vellus telogen* hair which is gradually shed.

573 Physiological alopecia Head rolling and friction produce hair loss on the back of the head. This disappears with development of stance.

574 Trichotillomania Patchy alopecia results from pulling and plucking ; a nervous tic in emotionally disturbed children.

575 Congenital baldness of the adult *androgenic* type seen in an abnormal baby with flexion deformity of the fingers (*see Patau and Edward's syndrome*).

572

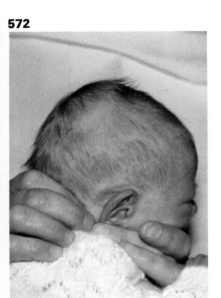

573

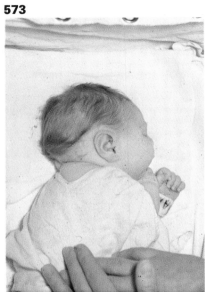

574

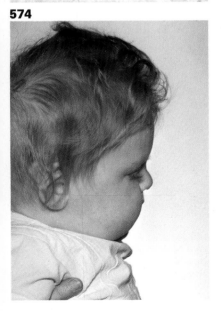

575

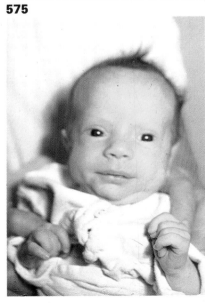

576 Congenital alopecia areata An ectodermal defect appearing over an atrophic skin.

577 Alopecia totalis A congenital familial disorder due to arrested development of hair follicles.

The 8-year-old girl had only a few strands of hair on the scalp. Eyebrows, eyelashes and body hair were missing. She had developed severe behaviour disorder, not alleviated by wearing an attractive wig.

576

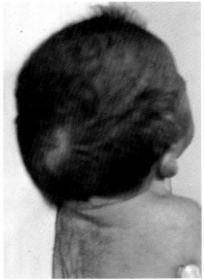

577

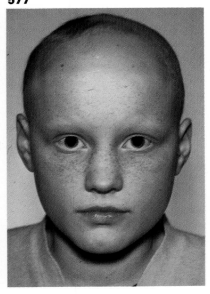

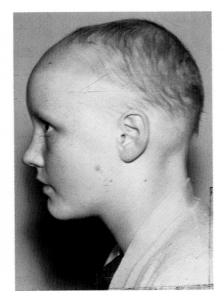

578 Hypertrichosis Newborn with a big tuft of hair forming a *cocks-crest* which cannot be smoothed down.

579 A similar case Abundant, unruly hair stands up over the entire scalp. Spasm of the erector pilorum in these hyperactive children is postulated.

580 Hirsutes situated on the upper part of the back and neck of this mentally defective child. The low hairline is shaped and confluent with the body hair.

578

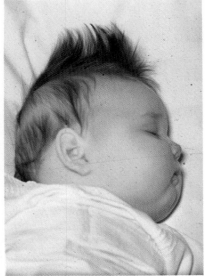

579

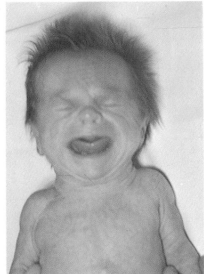

580

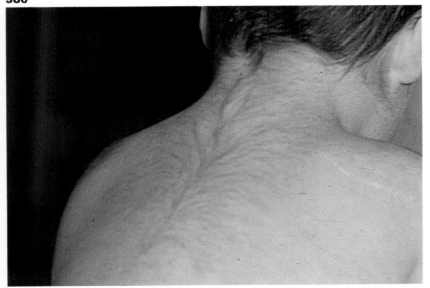

Idiopathic familial hypertrichosis (581-585) Increased sensitivity of hair follicles to normal levels of androgen is postulated.

581   At 4 years The boy has coarse features, pigeon chest, a muscular body, generalised hypertrichosis, abundant thick scalp hair with a shaped neckline and thick eyebrows and eyelashes. The penis and testicles are advanced for chronological age.

582 & 583   At 9 years Body build has improved. Hypertrichosis on the scalp and especially on the face has increased. Note the continuity of scalp hair with facial hair (**583**).

581

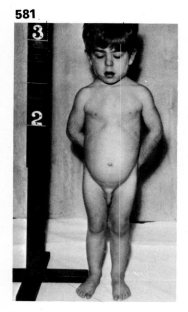
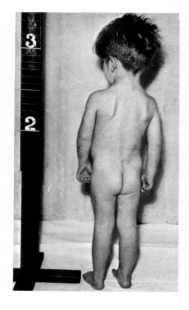

582

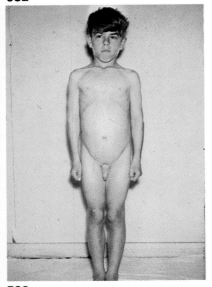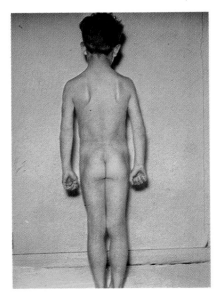

583

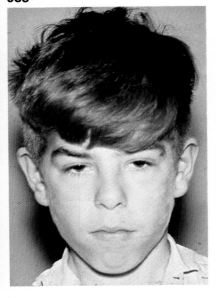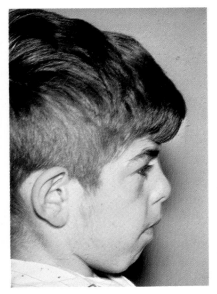

584 At 11 years, in puberty Hairiness has further increased, especially on the head, face and limbs. Bone age was advanced. The results of hormonal assay, nuclear sexing and chromosome analysis were those of a normal male. The father was of similar hairy appearance.

585 Another case The 8-year-old girl was not related, but had strikingly similar features. Nicknamed 'gorilla' by her schoolmates because of her hairiness, she developed schoolphobia.

584

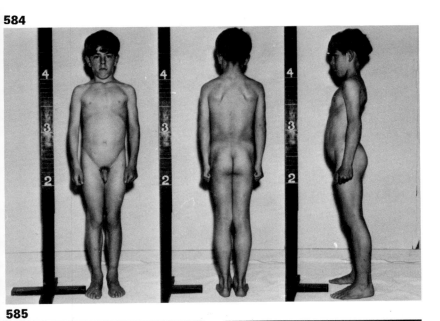

585

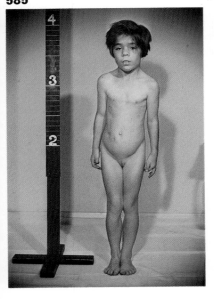

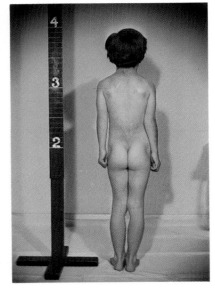

THE BATTERED CHILD SYNDROME (NON-ACCIDENTAL INJURY)

The syndrome defines recurrent physical injury, deprivation of nutrition, care and affection in young children motivated by a severely distorted parent-child relationship.

The clinical picture is bizarre, ranging from minor external injuries to multiple fractures in various stages of healing, and internal lesions occasionally with fatal outcome.

The diagnosis is difficult and not easily accepted. Organic disorders have to be excluded.

The rehabilitation of these children within the problem family is a complex legal and psycho-social procedure.

586 Assault The 18-month-old, illegitimate boy fell from a considerable height during 'play' with his mother. The colour of the periorbital ecchymoses and the left ptosis points to an old anterior fossa fracture. The fresh haemorrhagic bruises over the left temple indicate recent trauma.

586

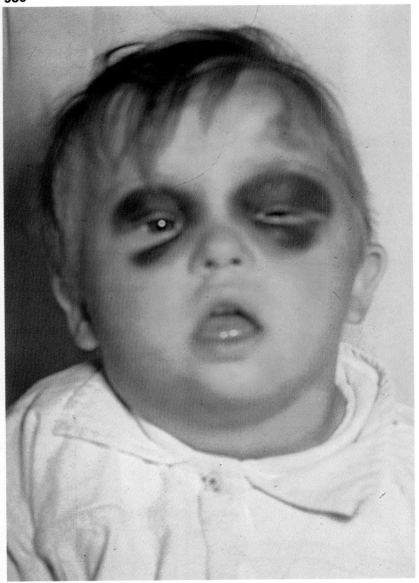

587 Another case The 6-year-old mongol came from a high social background. The resigned, forlorn attitude of the boy, the multiple bruises on the face and body, the swollen lips and dried crusts of blood around the nostrils testify to the assault.

588 Neglect This $2\frac{1}{2}$-year-old girl lived with foster parents. Note the expression of apathy and fear, the distended abdomen and signs of rickets on the thorax, wrists and ankles. Growth and intellectual milestones were delayed.

589 Malnutrition The 2-year-old was the unwanted youngest child of a large family. The pathetic, frightened expression and obvious signs of malnutrition resemble vitamin deficiencies and malabsorption. Note his attachment to a piece of soft material which he sucked whenever in distress.

590 One year later in residential care The physical condition has improved considerably. The emotional disturbance is still apparent. He clutches the same *amulet* as in the previous picture.

587

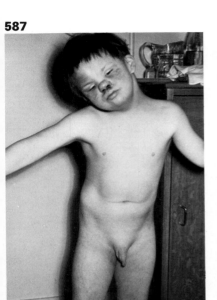

588

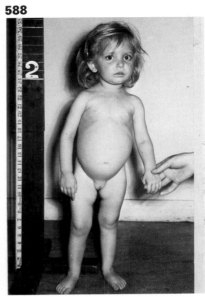

589

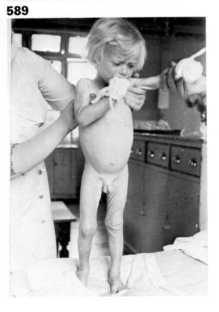

590

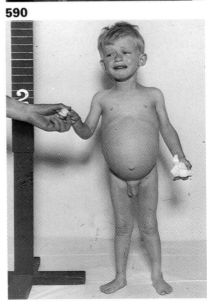

Tumours

591 A large pedunculated cyst is attached to the left toe.

592 Cavernous lymphangioma A common tumour, usually benign, but liable to infiltrate underlying structures and to recur after surgical removal.

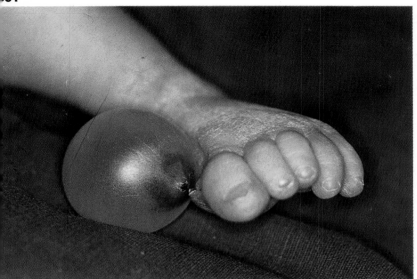

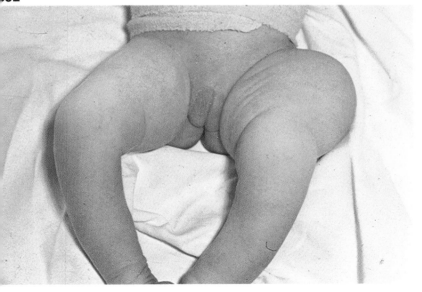

593-595 Cystic sublingual lymphangioma of the tongue in a 2-month-old infant. The tumour was present at birth and gradually grew to the size shown, causing surprisingly little breathing or feeding difficulties. The soft, spongy consistency allowed compression and temporary displacement of the cyst (**595**).

596 & 597 Appearance after aspiration and partial resection The prognathia of the lower jaw and the open mouth habit persisted.

593

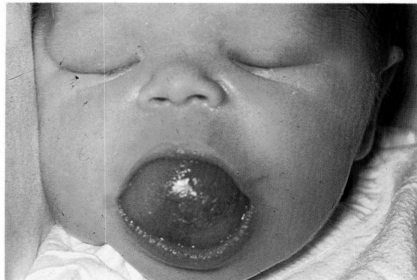

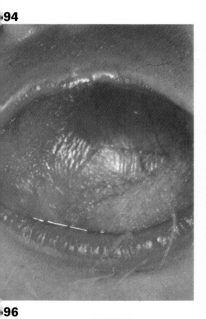

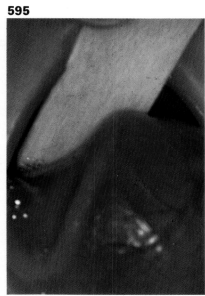

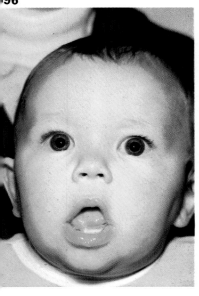

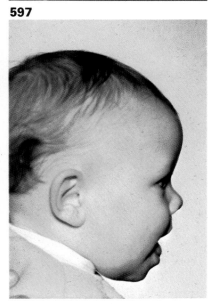

598 Hygroma colli A cystic lymphangioma with a tendency to rapid growth and extension into the mediastinum. Excision is imperative.

599 A pineal horn The growth was on the forehead, attached to the frontal bone above the nasal bridge, and was excised at the age of 10 days. Histology showed foci of ossification with newly formed bone cartilage and marrow in the subcutaneous tissue. Probably a hamartomous malformation.

600 At 1 year Marked hypertelorism, antimongolian slant of the palpebral fissures, and an alternating divergent squint have developed. Superfluous scar tissue with a bony core reached to the tip of the nose, which was everted.

601 & 602 At 3 years The peculiar disfiguration of the face has progressed. The scar was explored and a small cyst in the glabellar region was removed.

598

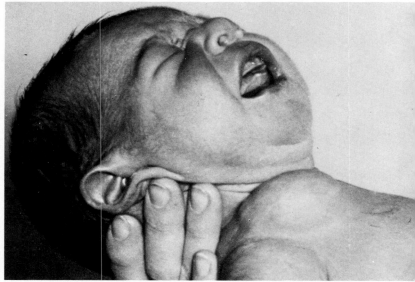

599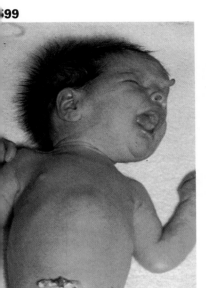

600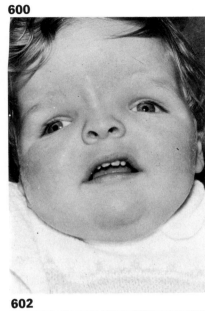

601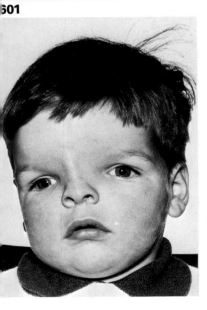

602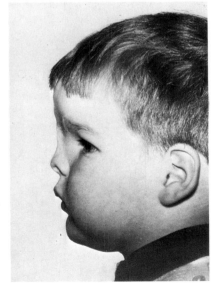

Neuroblastoma (603-606) The most common malignant tumour in early childhood. It originates in the adrenal area and along the sympathetic chain in the abdomen or chest, with a marked tendency to metastases throughout the body. The tumour is highly radio-sensitive. Spontaneous regression and maturation into a symptomless ganglioneuroma may occur.

603 Clinical picture. The 3-month-old girl suffered from restlessness, sweating and abdominal distension. Intravenous pyelography and abdominal x-ray revealed a large mass on the right side displacing the kidney downwards. Exploration and biopsy of the enormous liver showed mature liver tissue with multiple foci of neuroblastomas. Considered inoperable.

604 Vitamin B$_{12}$ treatment for 3 months. The liver regressed to normal size and abdominal circumference was reduced from 27 inches to 18$\frac{1}{2}$ inches. B$_{12}$ therapy was continued.

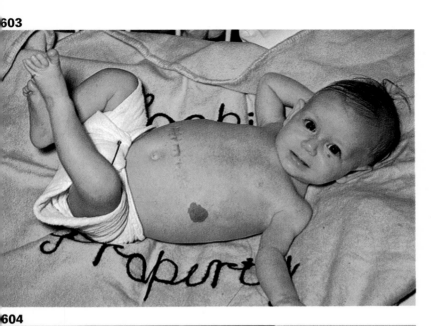

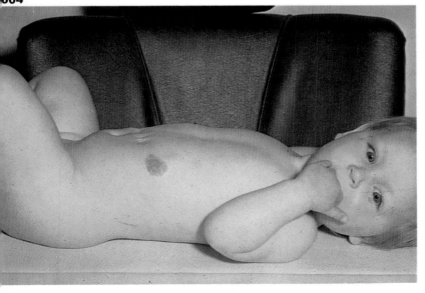

605 Same child at 2 years of age, in excellent health.

606 At 6 years she remained well. The value of B_{12} therapy is contro-versial considering the possibility of spontaneous regression.

607 Another case in an 8-year-old boy. Rapid progression of the large tumour and multiple skeletal metastases led to an early death.

605

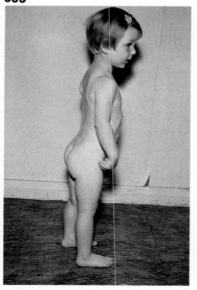
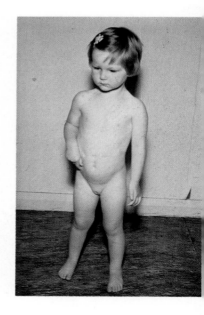

606

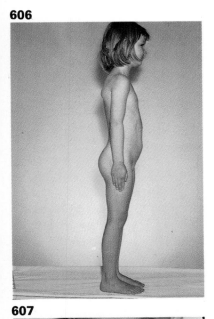 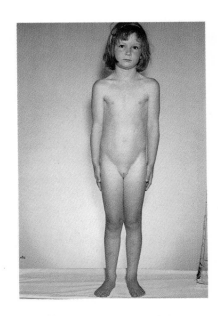

607

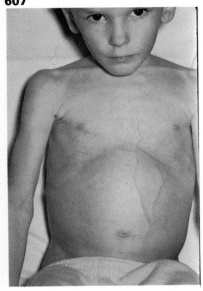 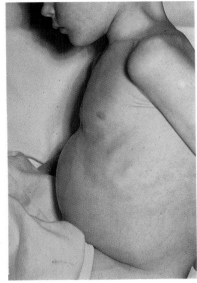

608-610 Congenital adenocarcinoma A very rare neoplasma. Widespread metastases into the skin and lungs were present at birth. The baby survived for 10 days.

608

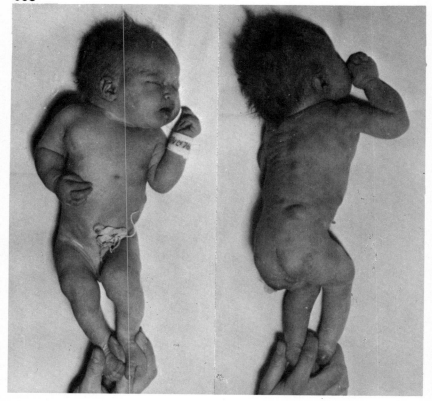

609

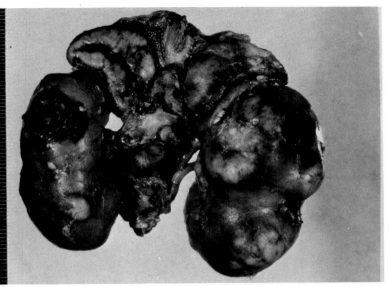

610

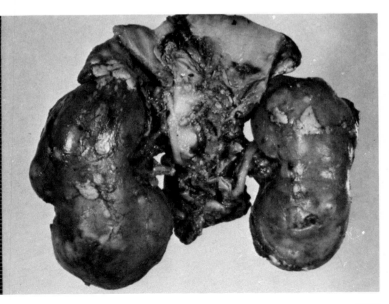

611 & 612 Carcinoma of the thyroid The 8-year-old boy had hoarseness and painless nodules in the neck. Note the deceptively satisfactory general condition. Biopsy revealed an anaplastic carcinoma of high malignancy. The boy died soon afterwards.

(*For other tumours see: lumbo-sacral teratoma,* **100***; adreno-cortical tumour,* **423-425***; granulosa cell tumour of the ovaries,* **426-427***; preauricular fibromas,* **435-438**)

611

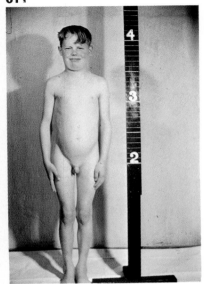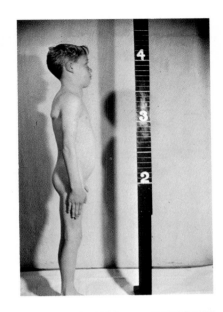

612

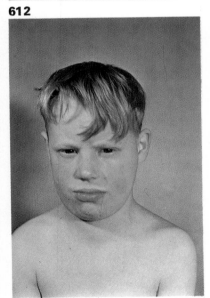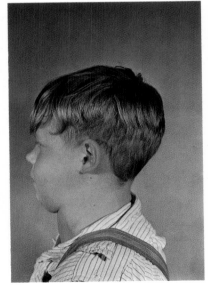

Miscellaneous

Minor anomalies are shown which though benign may simulate more serious conditions.

613 Lop-eared (bat-eared) 8-year-old boy Large flat auricles are protruding and bent forward because of missing antihelix folds ; a cosmetic defect which should be corrected before school age to avoid teasing.

614 White furred tongue caused by hypertrophy of filiform papillae during febrile conditions and dehydration.

615 Fissured (scrotal) tongue A congenital familial anomaly of obscure aetiology. The leaf-like or cerebriform pattern of the deep grooves is permanent, in contrast to the *geographical tongue* with its continuously changing pattern (*see* **326**).

613

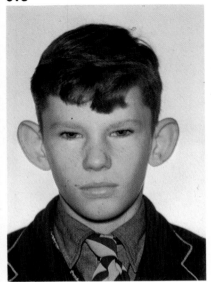

614

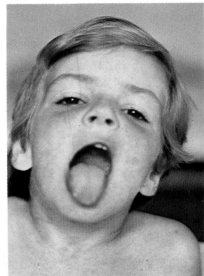

615

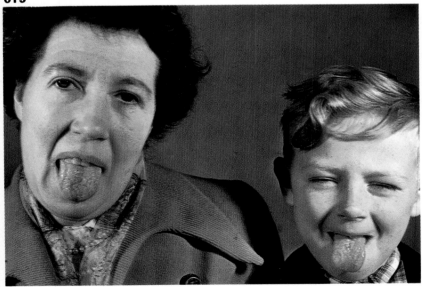

616 Stomatitis and thrush (monilia) Infection developed during prolonged antibiotic treatment.

617 Acne, seborrhoea and facial hypertrichosis A side effect of ACTH treatment, seen in a 3-month-old baby.

618 Accessory fingers and toes A minor anomaly; a *forme fruste* of polydactily, occasionally associated with other aberrations. More frequent in coloured children.

619 'Floppy child' syndrome, benign congenital hypotony (Walton) Muscular hypotonus and laxity of ligaments allow hypermobility of joints without discomfort. Improves gradually, but milestones are delayed. The diagnosis is one by exclusion (*see* **27, 28, 30, 458** *and* **459**).

616

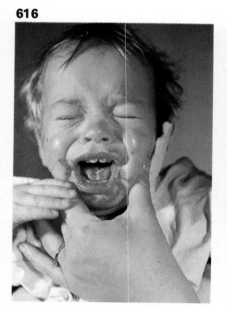

617

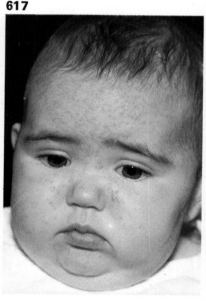

618

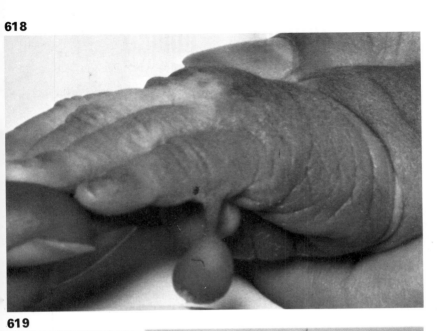

619

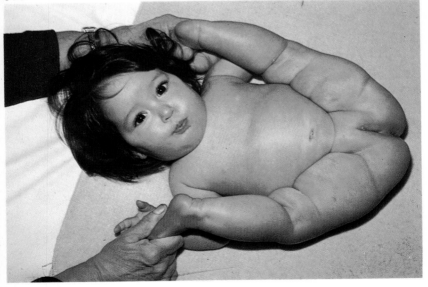

620 Pseudo-dysplasia of the hip joint Marked asymmetry of the thigh folds in the 4-month-old girl is suggestive of congenital dislocation of the hip. The backview shows the left gluteal fold higher than the right, but the crena ani is straight and the knee and ankle folds are symmetrical. The latter are diagnostic.

621 X-ray of the hip joint shows some shallowness of the acetabula which is of minor importance at this age.

622 Maximal abduction of the hip joint is equal and unlimited The *Ortolani jerk* of entry and exit is absent, thus excluding dislocation.
   This examination should be part of the screening programme of the newborn.

620

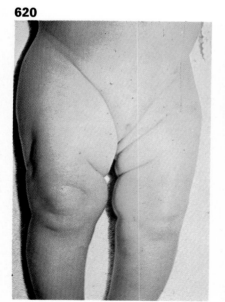 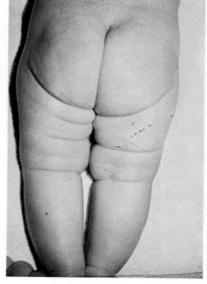

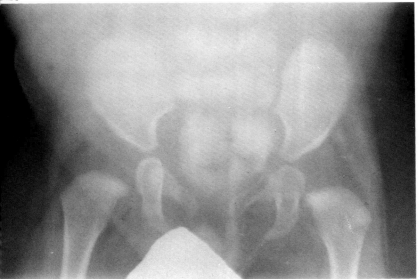

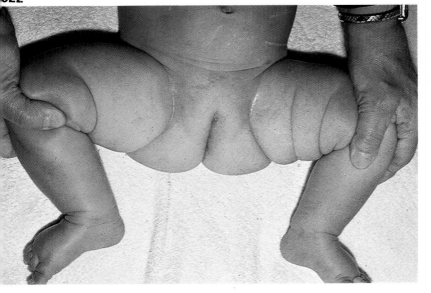

403

623 Synechia vulvae (adhesion of labia minora) The introitus is covered by a thin translucent membrane.

624 Treatment The membrane has been ruptured by gentle lateral traction. Application of oestrogen cream prevents recurrence. The condition, if overlooked, may lead to irritation and ascending infection.

625 Enlarged clitoris in a newborn There is normally some variability of size, but virilisation has to be excluded (*see* **233-234, 411-414**).

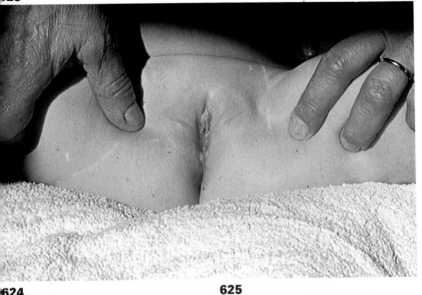

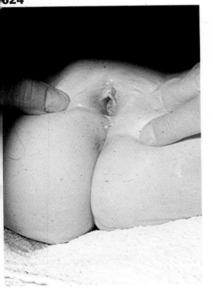

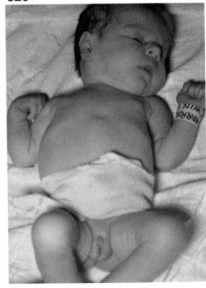

Appendix

FAECES

Inspection, analysis and bacteriology of faeces can give useful information about an infant's digestive function. Variations in consistency, frequency, colour and odour are indicative of specific disorders and stool analysis assists in the evaluation of absorption and possible enzyme defects.

626 Meconium The first stool passed within 36 hours after birth is preceded by the meconium plug. The greenish-black substance consists of swallowed hair, epithelial cells and intestinal secretion high in mucopolysaccharides. A high albumin content is found in cystic fibrosis, melaena and intestinal atresia.

627 The 'transition stool' shows the gradual change in colour and consistency with the introduction of milkfeeding (*first, second and fourth day, left to right*).

628 Breastmilk stools are golden-yellow, soft, slightly acid with small, soft fat and casein curds.

629 Cow's milk stools are pale yellow, pasty, homogenous, dry and alkaline, with numerous curds of calcium soaps.

626

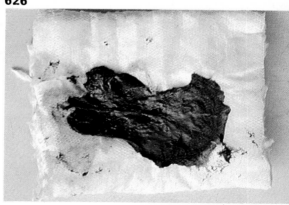

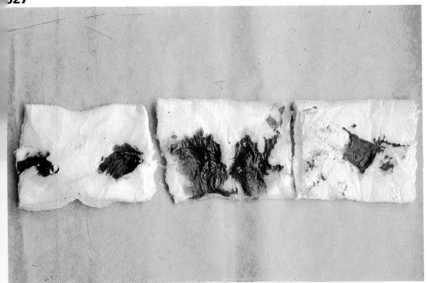

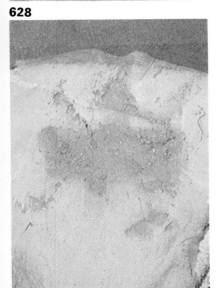

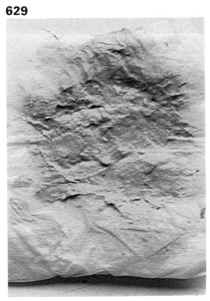

630 Green stools occur with intestinal hurry, or are due to oxidation of bilirubin to biliverdin by bacterial oxidation or when left exposed to air.

631 Mucoid green stools appear with intestinal irritation and peristaltic hurry during infection.

632 Acholic, pale stools contain colourless stercobilin due to lack of bile or incomplete reduction of bilirubin.

633 Red or black stools indicate the presence of blood from the lower or upper intestinal tract.

634 Scybalous, small stools result when breast feeding and fluid intake is insufficient.

630

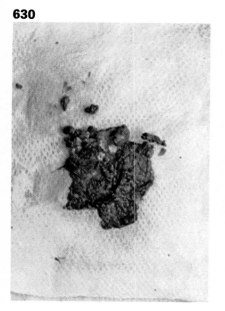

631

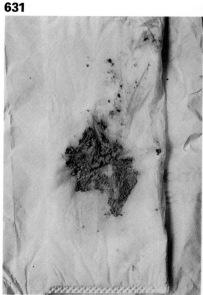

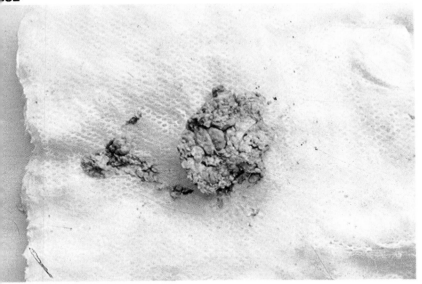

634

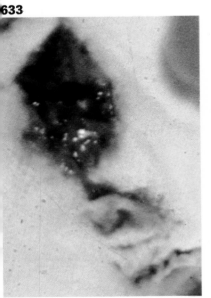

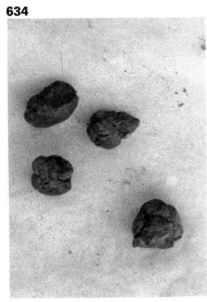

635 Pellet-like stools with artificial feeding are the result of undigested casein curds and calcium soaps, and of colonic spasm.

636 Bulky dark brown stools occur with constipation when an excess of protein and fat in the diet remains uncorrected by the addition of easily fermentable carbohydrates.

635

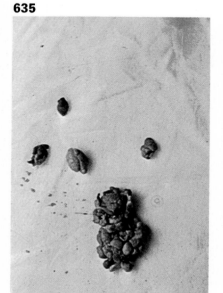

636

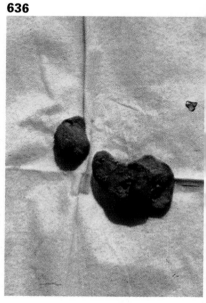

INDEX

413